JANELLE BEAUTY BOOK

Printed in the United States of America

First Printing, 2018

ISBN 978-0-578-40822-4

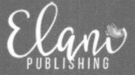

Elani Publishing
P.O. Box 2572, Forest VA 24551 USA
E-mail: info@elanipublishing.com
Website: www.elanipublishing.com

—

PHOTOGRAPHY

MICHAEL D SIMS   ANIKA J. PETTIFORD
SANDRA KIMBALL

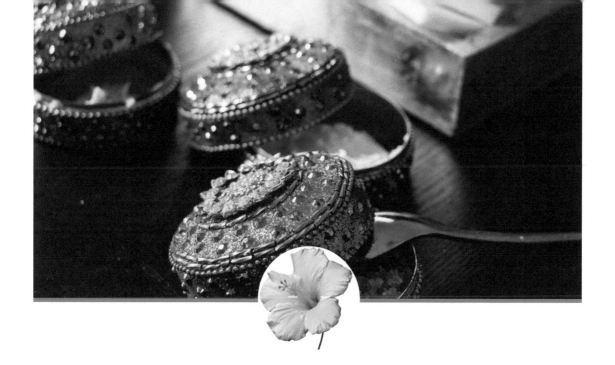

Dedication

This book is dedicated to my Lord and Savior Jesus Christ from whom all blessings flow. You spoke the word Lord, and it was so.

Thank you to my mom, Janet - the original Janelle Beauty and thank you to my daughter, Janelle - the next generation Janelle Beauty. Thank you to all my cousins and models who grace the pages of this book with your natural beauty! Your participation on this journey over the years has meant the world to me. I love you all!

Thank you to my brother Michael for helping me take my vision to the next level in the early days! I truly appreciate you! Thank you to all the Janelle Beauty staff, past & present for all their incredibly hard worrk!

Thank you to my husband Carl for letting me be who I am and allowing me to fly! I love you..

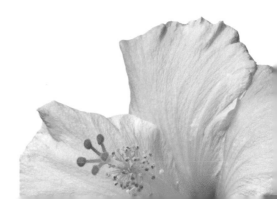

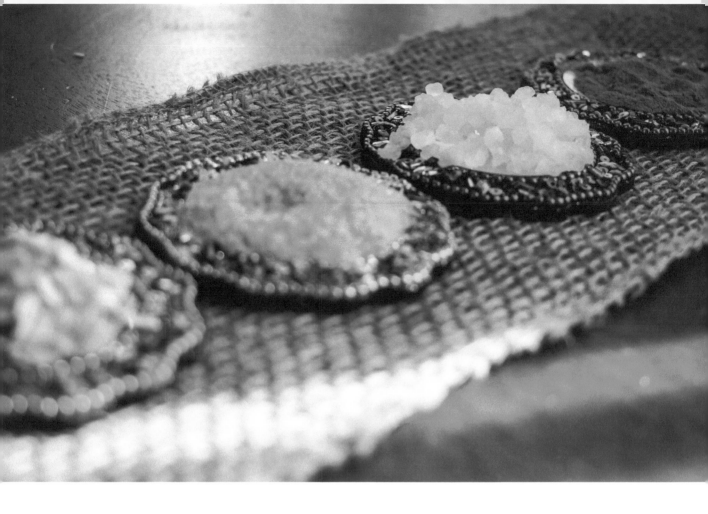

Contents BEAUTY RECIPES

Body: *skin loving recipes!*

Hair: *your crowning glory!*

Face: *get the glow!*

MEMOIR

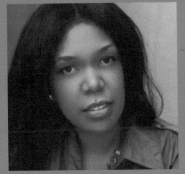

ANIKA JANELLE PETTIFORD

Founder & CEO

Follow the twists and turns of the tumultuous journey of Janelle Beauty the Brand. This short memoir is written in the words of company founder, Anika Janelle Pettiford

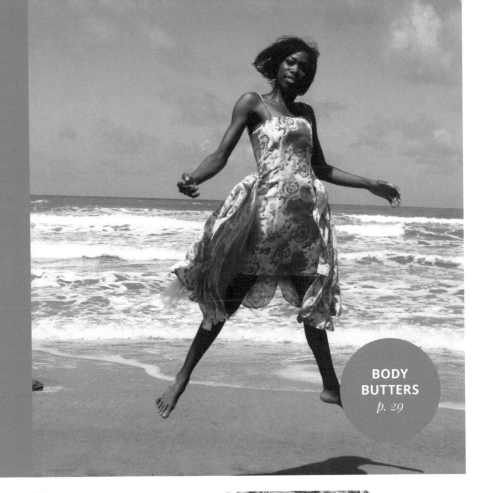

BODY BUTTERS
p. 29

TAME THE CURLS
p. 16

Janelle Beauty *the brand*

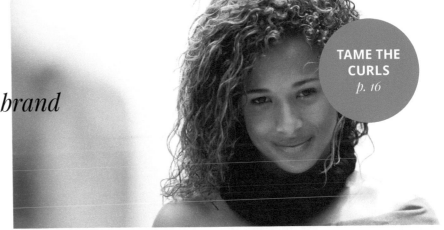

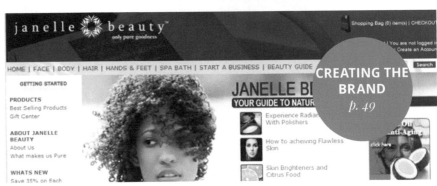

CREATING THE BRAND
p. 49

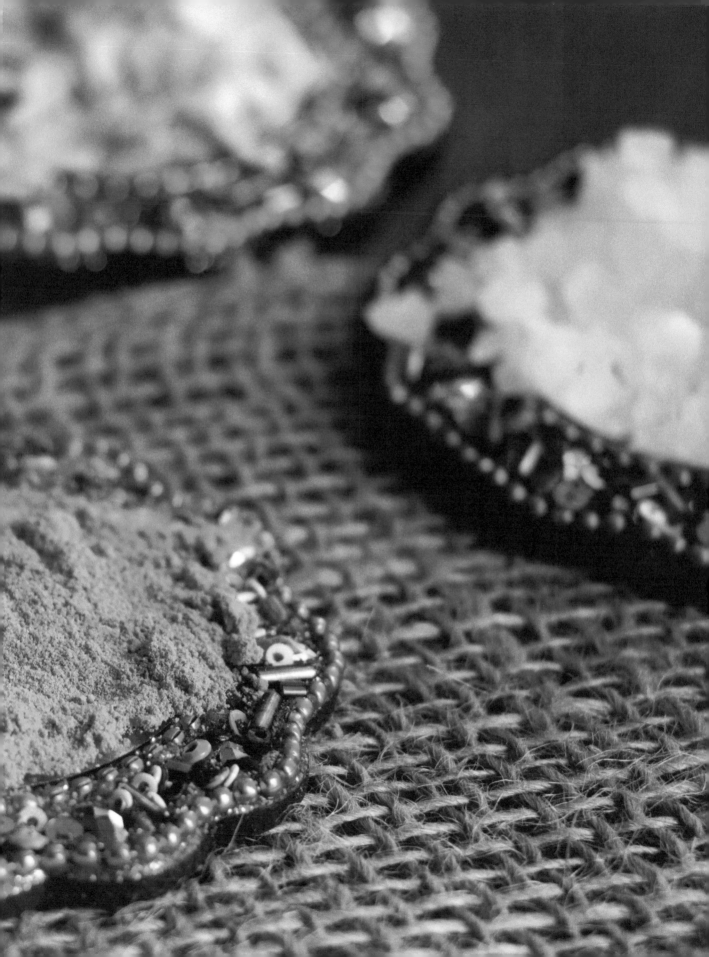

Beauty planner QUICK GUIDE

FLAWLESS *face*

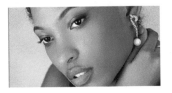

Grapeseed Facial Cream - For Oily Skin. **P. 42**

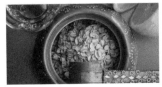

Honey & Oats Facial Scrub. **P. 47**

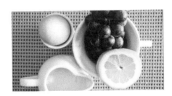

Grape & Milk Facial Mask. **P. 69** ● ●

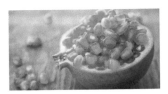

Pomegranate Facial Cream. **P. 52**

AT HOME *spa*

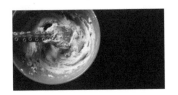

Chocolate Almond Body Butter. **P. 32**

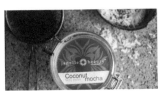

Coconut Mocha Body Polish **P. 39** ● ● ●

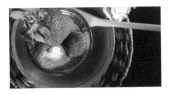

Strawberry Body Buttr Scrub. **P. 51**

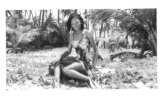

Ginger Bath Salts. **P. 59**

MY NATURAL *curl*

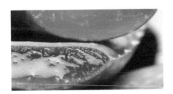

Aloe Hair Rub. **P. 15** ● ●

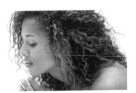

Oats & Honey Deep Conditioning Treatmet. **P. 23**

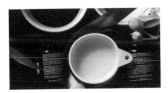

Smoothie For Curls **P. 17** ● ●

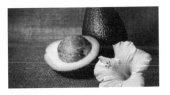

Avocado Mask. **P. 23**

WEAR IT *smooth & straight*

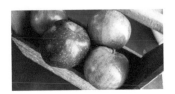

Smoothing Hair Rinse. **P. 22**

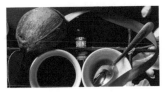

Honey & Molasses Hair Smoothie. **P. 20** ● ● ●

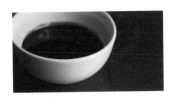

Molasses Mask. **P. 19**

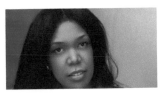

My Journey to Natural Hair **P. 11**

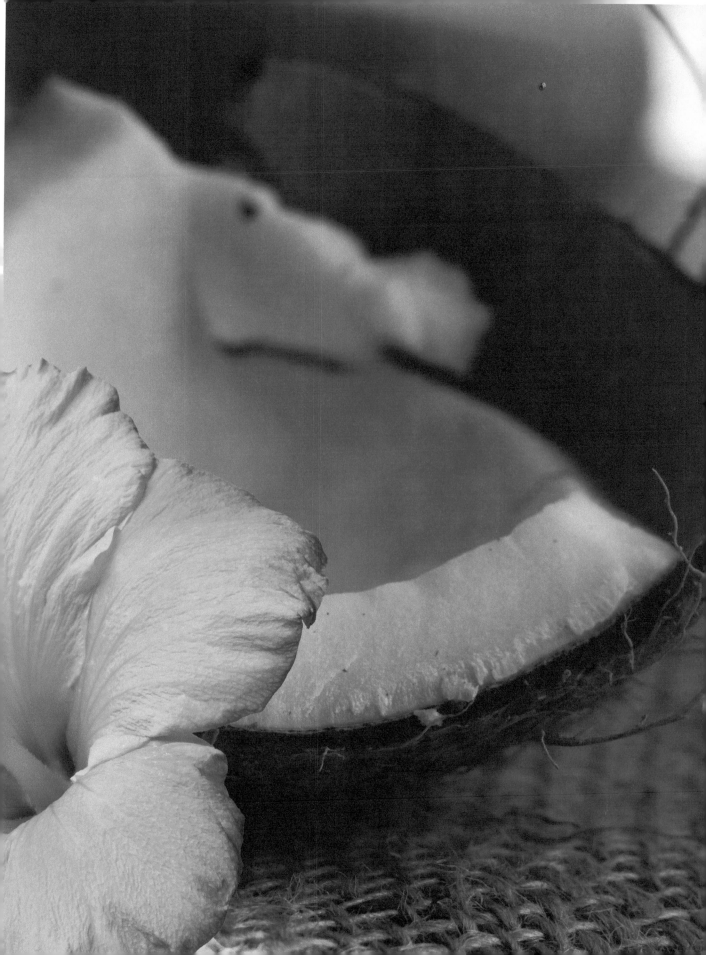

GENESIS: A Vision is Born

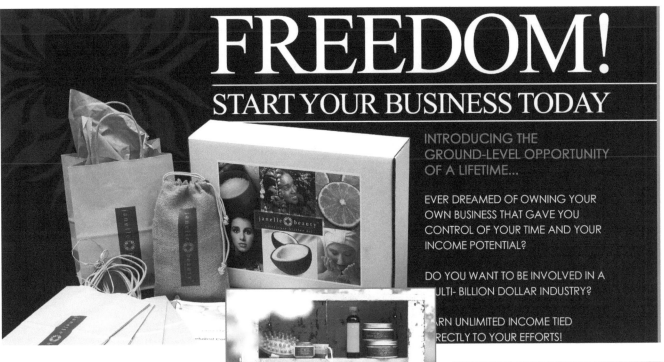

FREEDOM!
START YOUR BUSINESS TODAY

INTRODUCING THE
GROUND-LEVEL OPPORTUNITY
OF A LIFETIME...

EVER DREAMED OF OWNING YOUR
OWN BUSINESS THAT GAVE YOU
CONTROL OF YOUR TIME AND YOUR
INCOME POTENTIAL?

DO YOU WANT TO BE INVOLVED IN A
MULTI- BILLION DOLLAR INDUSTRY?

EARN UNLIMITED INCOME TIED
DIRECTLY TO YOUR EFFORTS!

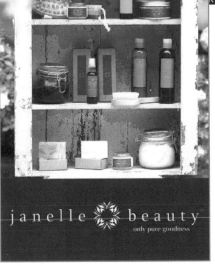

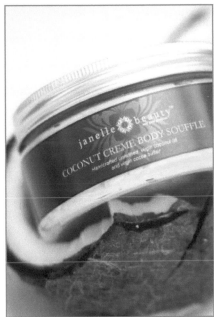

Once upon a time

It is said that necessity is the mother of invention and that is exactly what led to the conception of Janelle Beauty. It was not in my life plan to start a beauty company. It was not even a thought on my mind. It was born out of necessity and a gap in the market for the products I needed.

My life was interrupted by an ailment that led me on a journey to health and wholeness. That journey led to a new world of beauty products that quickly got complicated when my focus turned to my hair.

As a woman of color, finding the right products that were 1. Efficacious and 2. High-quality was no easy feat.

However, I was determined to get what I needed even if it meant creating it myself. And that in a nutshell, was how Janelle Beauty was born.

MEMOIR: *what do i do* **Now!**
It all began with HAIR
Why do your beauty products matter to your health?
The solution - eat well and make your own beauty care creations!

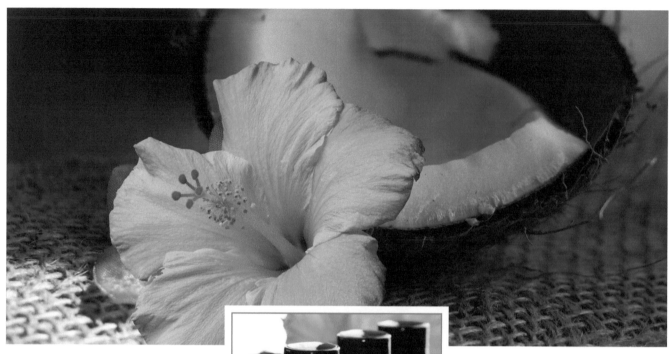

After getting my diagnosis, I left the doctor's office in a daze. What does this mean? Of course ,I had to research and figure out exactly what I was dealing with. After my initial research, it did not look good. And as we all know now, never go to the internet to find out what is wrong with you. By the time I was done, I just knew that I was going to die!

With tears in my eyes, I continued researching and bought books and attended seminars and one thing led to another and the next thing I knew, my diet was radically changed and then my attention was suddenly turned to my skincare and beauty products.

I started realizing things I never thought about in my life. Things like the fact that your skin is the largest organ in your body and it actually absorbs what you rub into and lather on it. That was obvious yet startling! The question then became, is what I am using on my skin good enough to enter into my body?

If a birth control patch can affect my reproductive system; what else in my body can be affected by the lotions, potions, shampoos and conditioners I use on my body everyday?
My research continued and it was not looking good. In the meantime, I decided to throw out all my beauty care products.

My diet was coming along well and my health had vastly improved. But I had a serious beauty problem. I was like a cavewoman. No shampoo, No conditioner, no lotions, no chemical relaxers, no styling products, no nothing! It was time to make my own beauty treasures. It was the only way to ensure my products were filled with ONLY PURE GOODNESS! I attacked my hair problem first. After all, it's all about the hair!

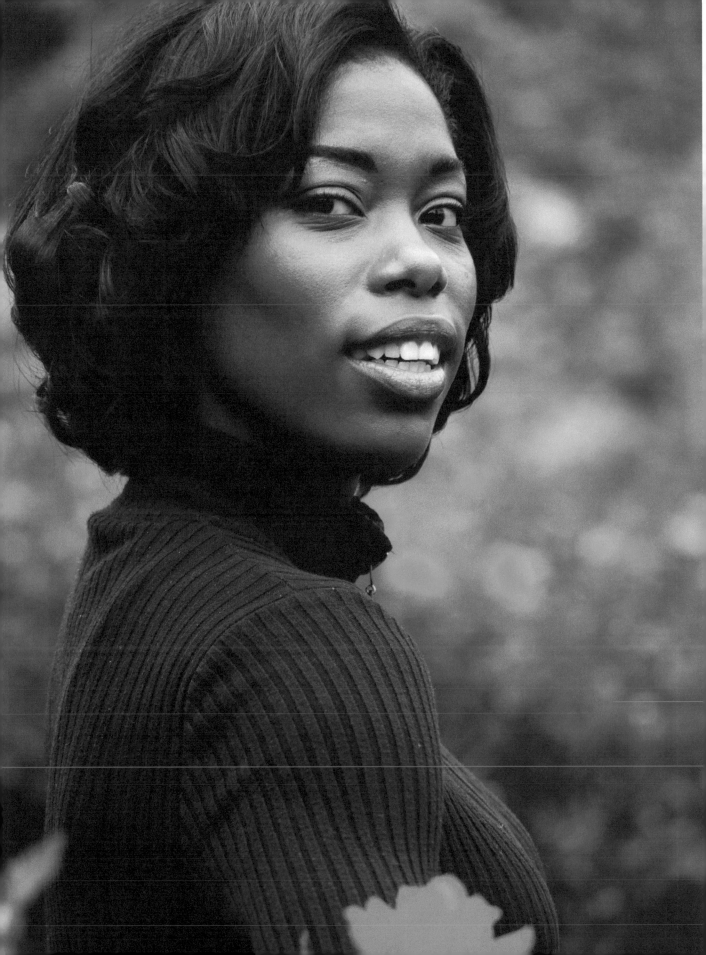

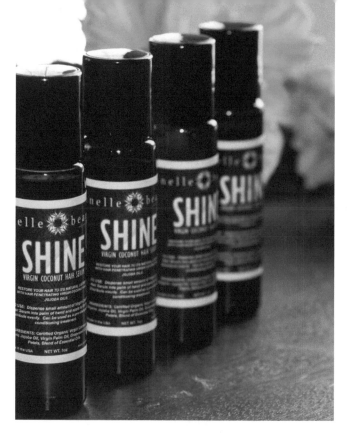

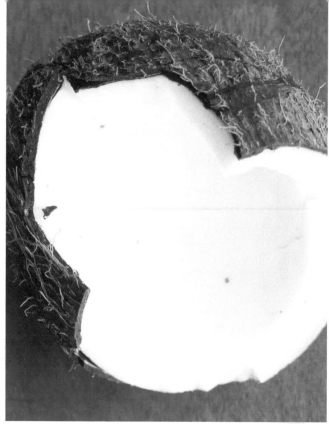

JOURNEY
to natural hair

The first casualty in my quest to natural living and using natural beauty products was my regularly scheduled chemical relaxer.

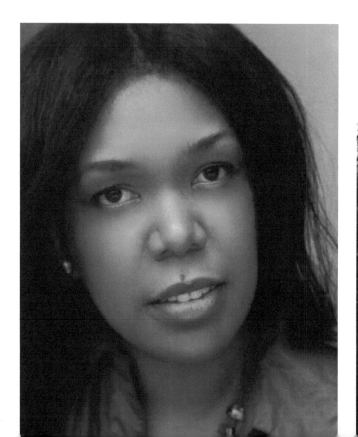

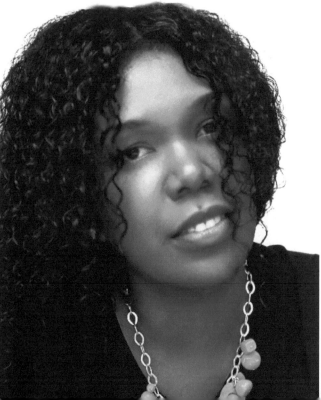

KEY INGREDIENT BENEFIT LIST

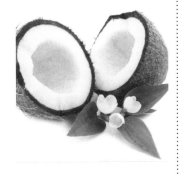

Jojoba Oil - Organic - The molecular structure of jojoba is very similar to the natural oil that is produced by the sebaceous glands in the scalp known as sebum. It is a well-known fact that sebum is required in maintaining healthy supple hair. Hair that has a good moisture basis tends to be more resistant to daily damage, tangles. dryness and split ends. Jojoba oil comes from the jojoba plant.

straight linear chain, it is able to penetrate the hair shaft.

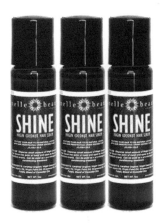

Virgin Coconut Oil
Reduces the protein loss for both undamaged and damaged hair. Coconut oil, being a triglyceride of lauric acid (principal folly acid), has a high affinity for hair proteins. Because of its low molecular weight and

MEMOIR: MY JOURNEY TO NATURAL HAIR

The first casualty in my quest to natural living and natural beauty products was my regularly scheduled chemical relaxer. I did not do the big chop that most women do when they make this momentus decision. I decided to grow out my relaxer. This left me with kinky-curly roots and straight ends. I needed a solution to facilitate a smooth transition to naturally curly tresses. My quest led me to the oil of the coconut.

Growing up in Trinidad, coconuts were an integral part of my life. The trees swaying in the wind is an indelible picture of my child-hood. When I found out that the main fatty acid found in coconut oil has the ability to penetrate the hair shaft, I was intrigued. I also discovered that the oil, when applied with heat via a flat-iron, can actually coat the hair naturally and give you a smooth, straight finish.

This was my solution! I created my own signature concoction and made my transition to natural hair seamlessly.

I propose that you try making your own natural solutions so that you have the absolute guarentee that your are only using the best and finest natural ingredients. If you want the second best option - shop Janelle Beauty!

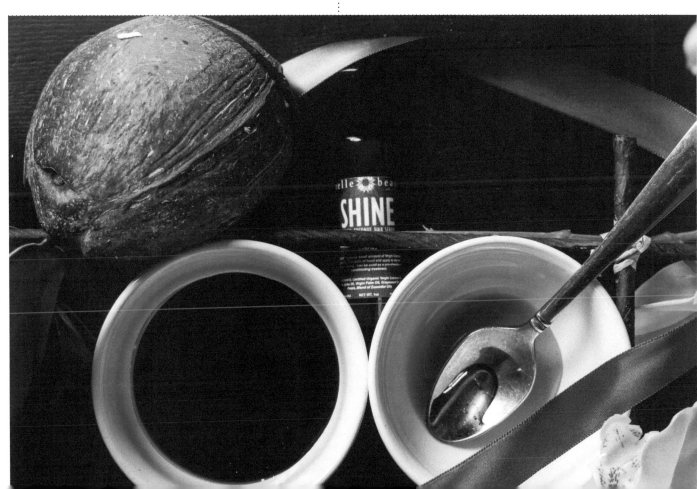

THE WONDERS OF HONEY

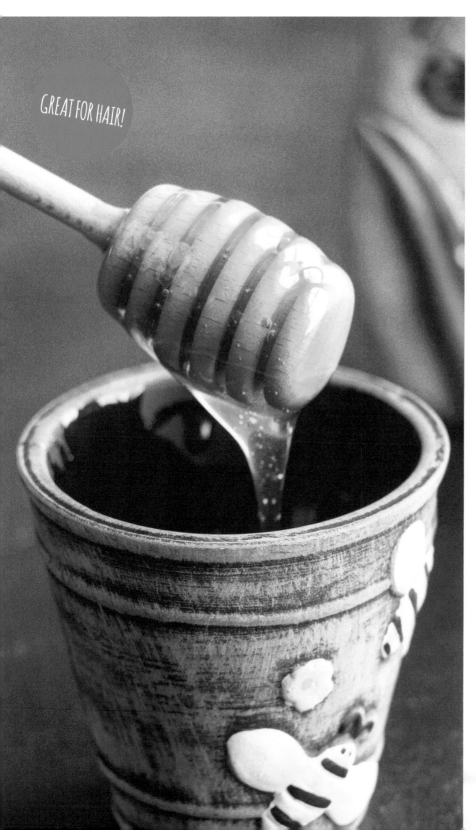

GREAT FOR HAIR!

Honey is known for its many benefits when used on the hair and skin. honey is a humectant, which makes it an excellent moisturizing ingredient in hair and face tonics.

THREE AMAZING BENEFITS OF HONEY:

1 **Honey is rich in natural anti-oxidants and have anti-micro-bial properties.**

2 **Honey also has the ability to absorb and retain mois-ture.** This helps in keeping the skin well hydrated, fresh and supple..

3 **Honey restores dry, dam-aged and dull-looking hair.** It helps retain moisture and get rid of dry, itchy flakes on your scalp.

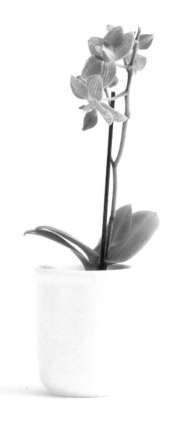

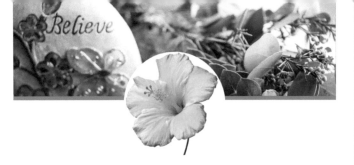

BEAUTY SECRET

Aloe Hair Rub

Inside the hard skin of the aloe leaf is a highly prized treasure. The gel like substance is exploding with only pure goodness for your hair!

Here is a simple recipe to add ridiculous moisture and shine to natural hair. The enzymes help both the scalp and the hair lock in moisture.

Aloe leaf 1

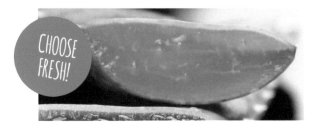

CHOOSE FRESH!

1   Part hair into 4 sections.

2   Cut aloe leaf into 4 pieces and remove the outer skin. Take the gel like substance and rub into each section of parted hair. Apply from scalp to ends until whole head is covered.

3   Let sit for 30 minutes.

4   Rinse and apply conditioner. Style as usual.

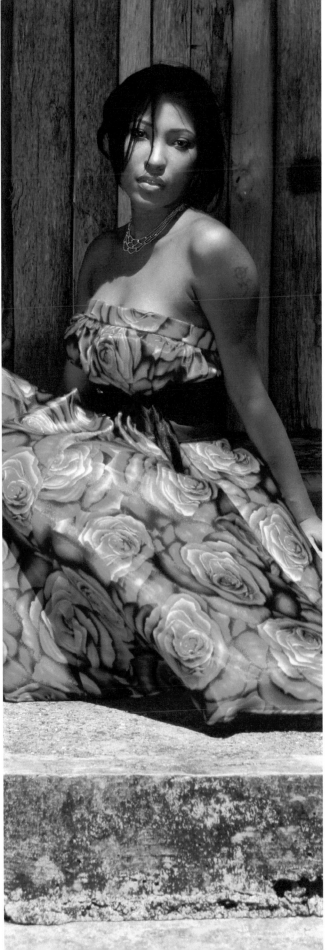

TAME THE CURLS

Curly hair is such a blessing! However, as a recipient of this particular blessing I can sometimes be unappreciative when I have to tame my curls to the look I desire for the day. Sometimes I let my curls do what they want to do and call it a day! Other times I want to define my curls to get that certain look. It's all about options!

CURLY HAIR

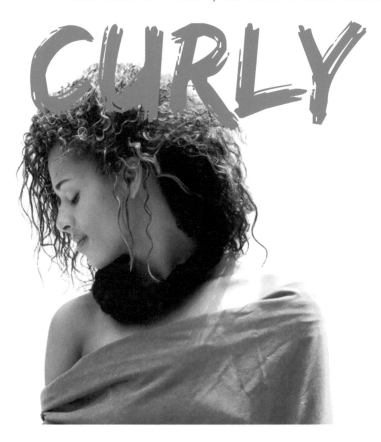

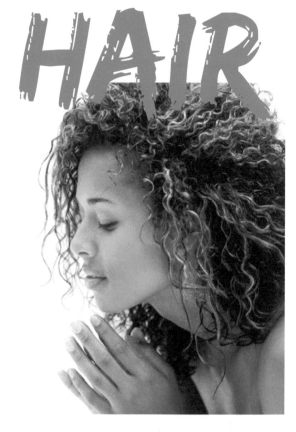

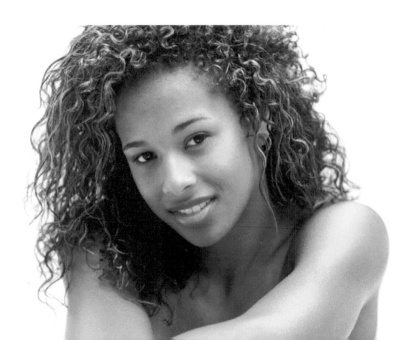

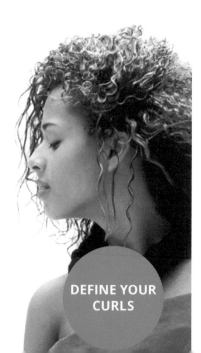

DEFINE YOUR CURLS

Mix *like a* **Pro Artisan!**
SMOOTHIE FOR CURLS

Super ingredient Molasses makes an appearance in this smoothie for curls.

Tip: Apple cider vinegar gives incredible shine.

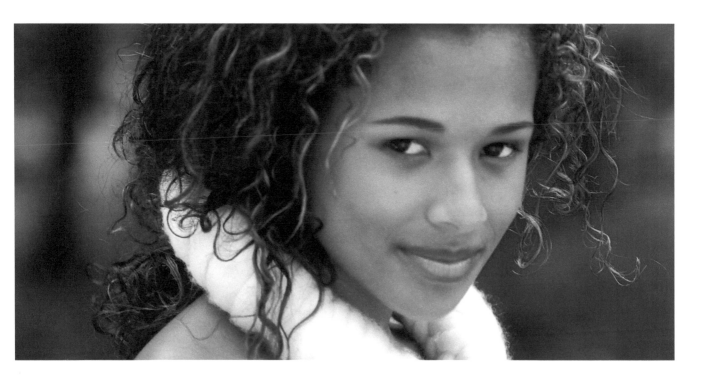

Smoothie for Curls

Molasses 2 ozs
Lemon Juice 2 tbsp
Apple Cider Vinegar 2 tbsp
Corn Starch 1 tbsp
Olive Oil 2 tbsp
Argan Oil 1 tbsp
Essential oils 5 drops

1   Mix all ingredients in bowl with an electric mixer.

2   Apply with fingers over dry or wet hair, from roots to ends.

3   Leave on for 30 minutes.

4   Rinse and Shampoo, then apply Conditioner.

5   Rinse and style your curls.

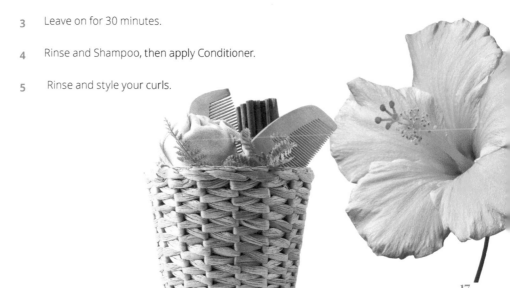

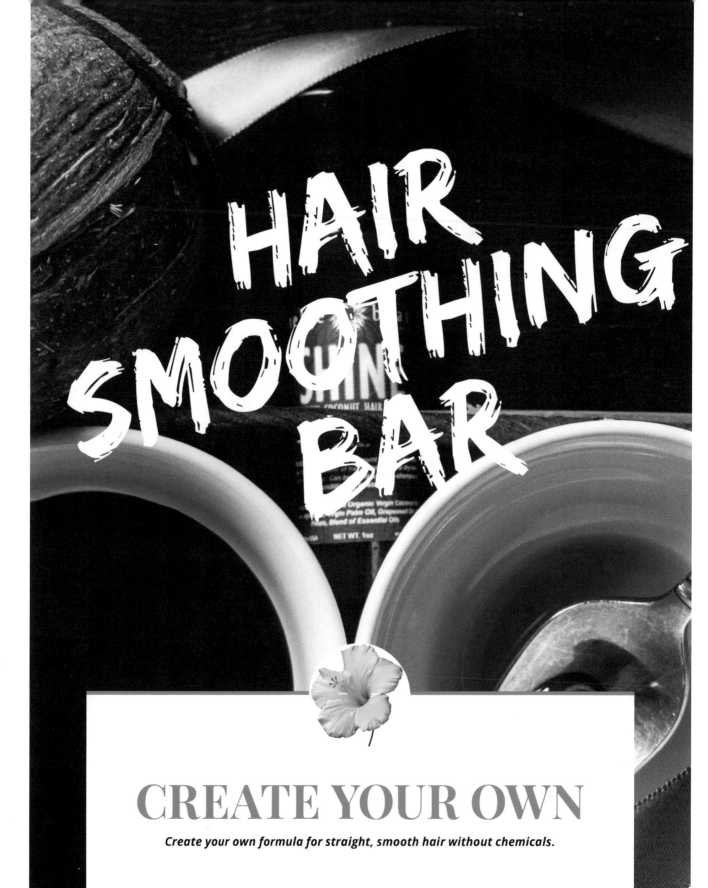

CREATE YOUR OWN

Create your own formula for straight, smooth hair without chemicals.

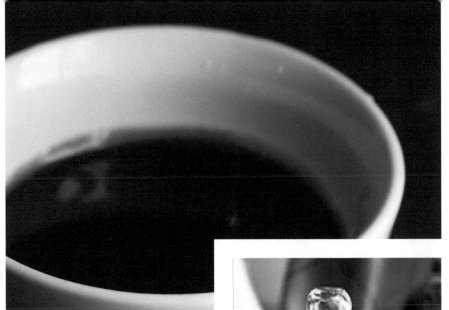

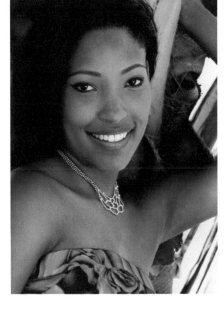

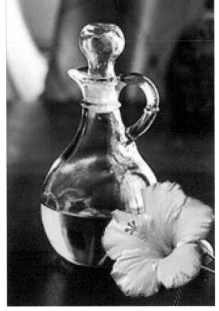

MOLASSES HAIR MASK

Molasses 4 tbsps
Water 1 tbsp
Argan oil 1 tsp

1. Mix to desired consistency and apply to hair. Leave on hair for 20 minutes and then rinse. Apply conditioner and proceed with your regular regimen.

THE POWER OF MOLASSES

Blackstrap molasses is what i call a super-power hair food! It is loaded with antioxidants and it is high in vitamins and minerals; more specifically, trace minerals that your hair craves. Molasses is a double-edged sword for those combating dry, damaged hair since its benefits can be gleaned by ingestion and topical application.

High amounts of potassiun, manganese, copper, iron, vitamin B6 etc can be found in this power hair food. There are a lot of testimonials affirming the amazing benefits of molasses, including hair growth, fuller hair and even fighting gray hair!

The major reason molasses should be one of your main ingredients in your hair smoothie is the high deposit of moisture applied to your hair. Shiny smooth tresses are the result of this powerful ingredient in your hair concoctions whether straight or curly.

You can add molasses to your hair smoothie recipes, or you can use it as a stand alone hair mask after you shampoo and before you apply conditioner.

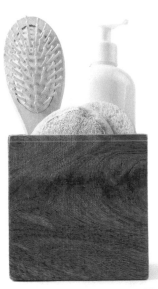

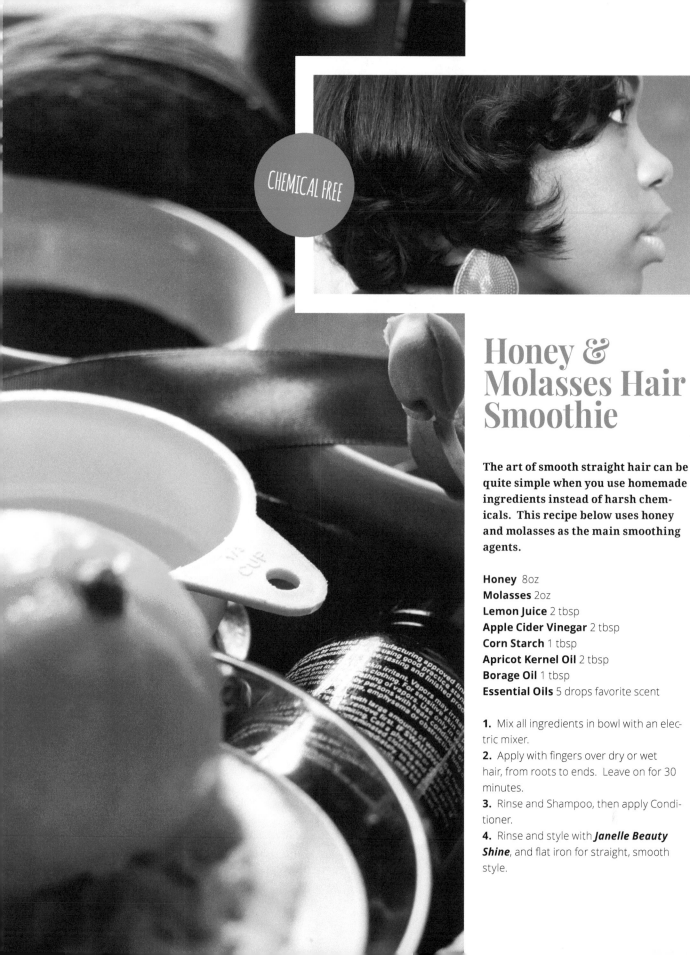

Honey & Molasses Hair Smoothie

The art of smooth straight hair can be quite simple when you use homemade ingredients instead of harsh chemicals. This recipe below uses honey and molasses as the main smoothing agents.

Honey 8oz
Molasses 2oz
Lemon Juice 2 tbsp
Apple Cider Vinegar 2 tbsp
Corn Starch 1 tbsp
Apricot Kernel Oil 2 tbsp
Borage Oil 1 tbsp
Essential Oils 5 drops favorite scent

1. Mix all ingredients in bowl with an electric mixer.
2. Apply with fingers over dry or wet hair, from roots to ends. Leave on for 30 minutes.
3. Rinse and Shampoo, then apply Conditioner.
4. Rinse and style with *Janelle Beauty Shine*, and flat iron for straight, smooth style.

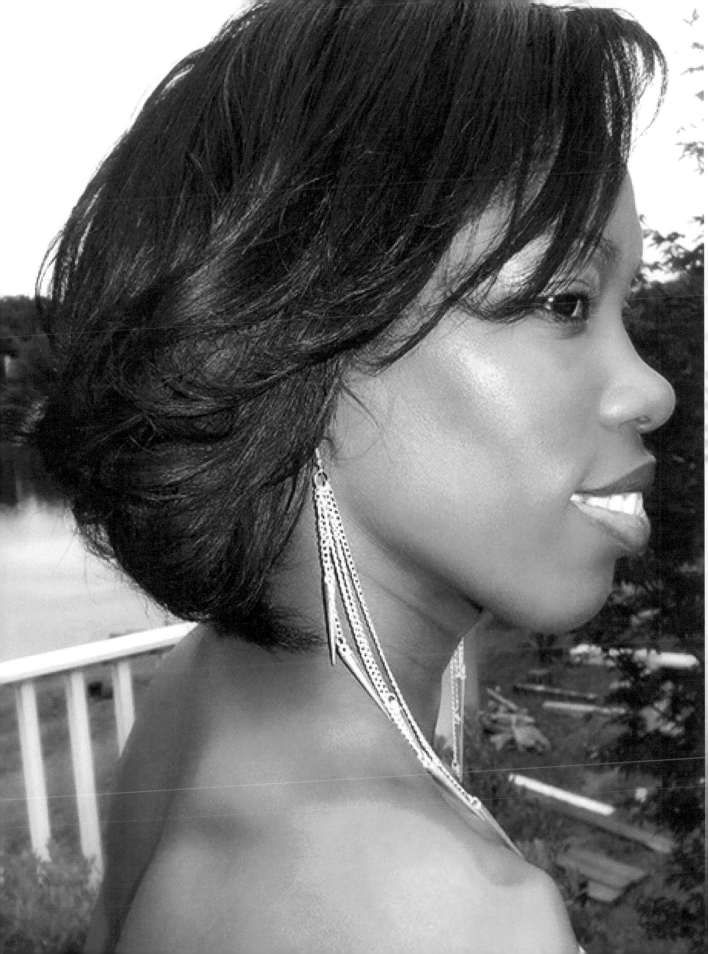

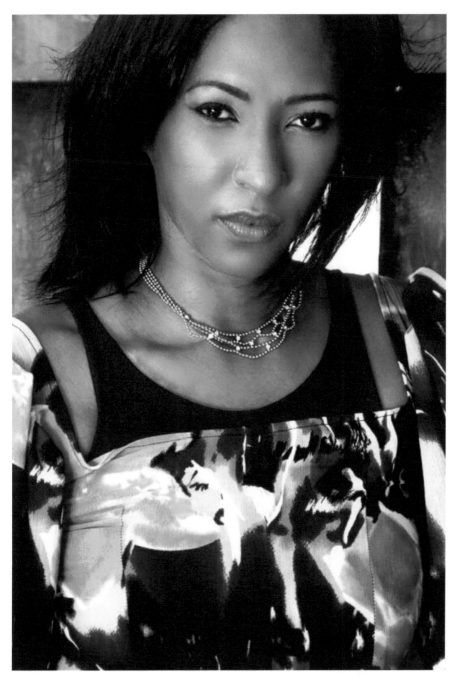

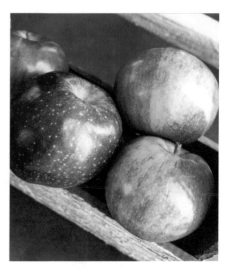

This hair rinse can be used after you've applied and rinsed out your shampoo and just before you apply conditioner. This Smoothing Hair Rinse will seal the hair cuticle and coat hair with an incredible shine!

"Shiny, bouncy hair"

Mix 4 ozs of Apple cider vinegar with 4 ozs of warm water and you are done! Apply to hair and leave on for a few minutes and rinse. Apply conditioner.

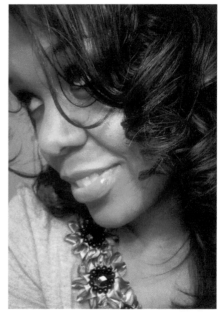

Smoothing *Hair Rinse*

Apple cider vinegar is one of the wonders of the natural hair world! Its benefits are numerous, and its results are optimal.

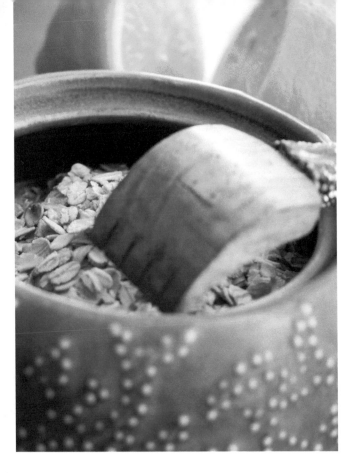

Honey & Oats Deep Conditioning Treatment

Cooked oatmeal 1 cup
Raw honey 1 tbsp
Jojoba oil 1 tsp
Your favorite **essential oil*** to scent, 2 drops

1. Mix all ingredients until smooth.

2. Part hair into 4 sections.

3. Apply to hair, root to ends until complete coverage.

4. Leave on for at least 20 minutes and rinse. Apply conditioner. Style as desired.

*Essential oils are highly potent and should be used with care. Follow all safety precautions from manufacturer when using essential oils. Please consult physician before extensive use of essential oils.

Avocado Hair Mask

Avocado 1 mashed
Lemon juice 1 tsp
Jojoba oil 2 tsp
Your favorite **essential oil*** to scent, 2 drops

1. Mix all ingredients until smooth.

2. Part hair into 4 sections.

3. Apply to hair, root to ends until complete coverage.

4. Leave on for at least 20 minutes and rinse. Apply conditioner. Style as desired.

*Essential oils are highly potent and should be used with care.

Follow all safety precautions from manufacturer when using essential oils. Please consult physician before extensive use of essential oils.

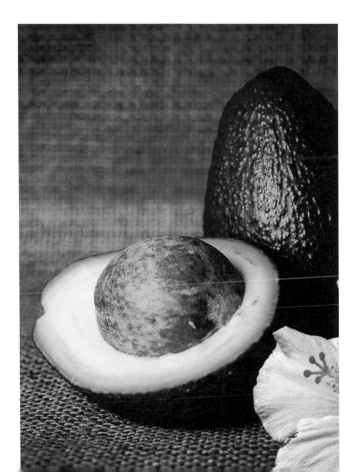

MEMOIR

His
grace abounds to me

My journey up to this point in creating my own beauty treasures was all about me. The year was 2005 and I was getting really deep into this "creating my own cosmetic thing." I played around with so many recipes and ingredients and I moved past hair care into creating body care products. The following pages are full of recipes that I worked on over the years. I hope you enjoy them as much as I enjoyed making them!

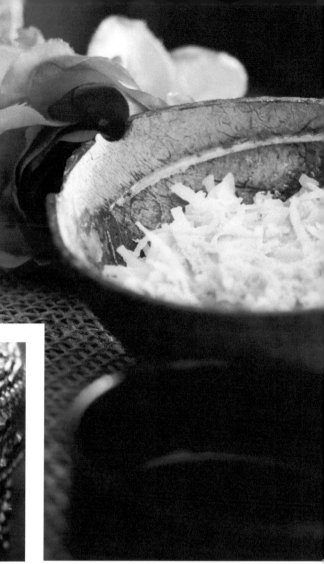

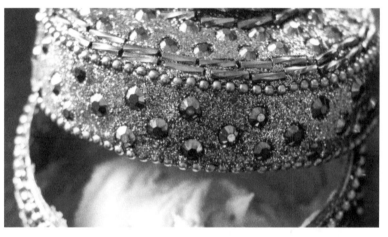

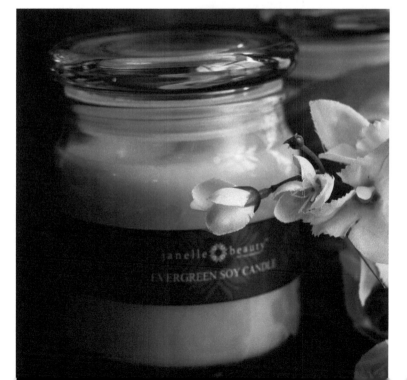

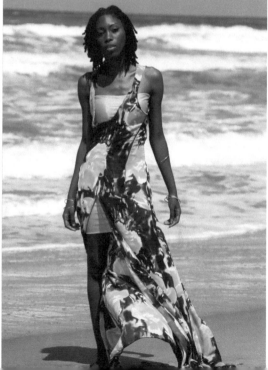

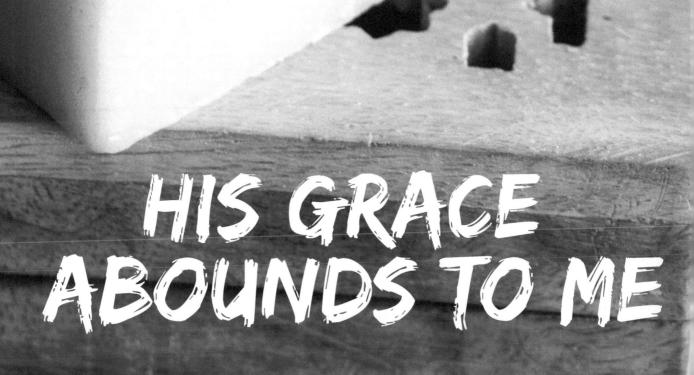

HIS GRACE
ABOUNDS TO ME

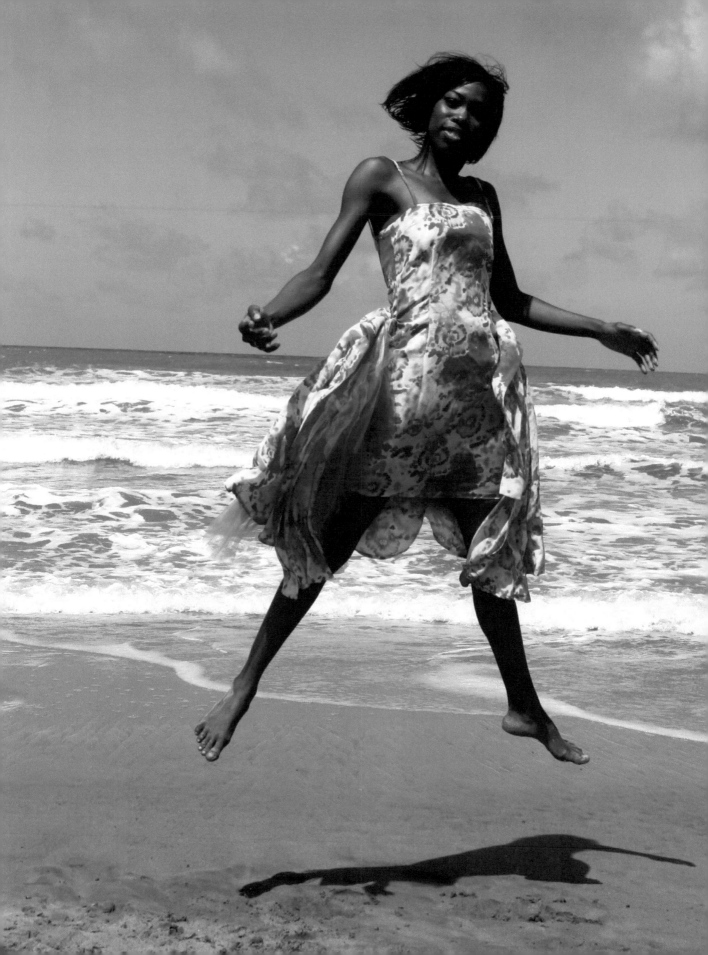

Pink Grapefruit Sugar Scrub

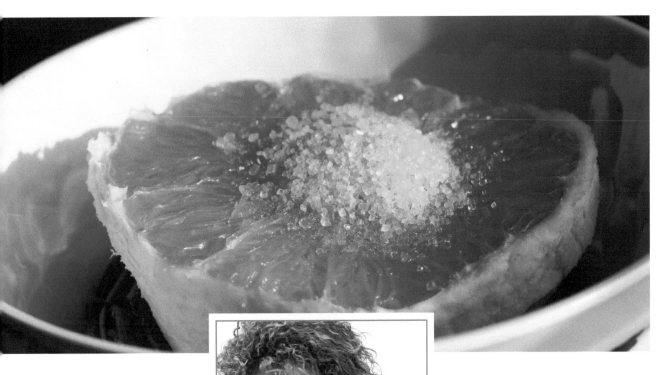

Half a **grapefruit**
Sugar 1 tbsp
Jojoba oil 1 tsb

1. Combine the sugar and oil.
2. Squeeze a bit of the grape-fruit juice into the sugar and oil mixture.
3. Scoop the mixture into the center of grapefruit.
4. On wet skin use the filled grapefruit as a loofah and scrub hardened skin areas first. Rinse.

BENEFITS OF GRAPEFRUIT

The antioxidant and vitamin dense grapefruit is an excellent loofah to slough off dead skin cells and even skin tone.

The benefits of grapefruit are too numerous to mention but suffice it to say that the Vitamins A and C found in grapefruit promotes healthy, glowing skin!

Let *your skin* shine!

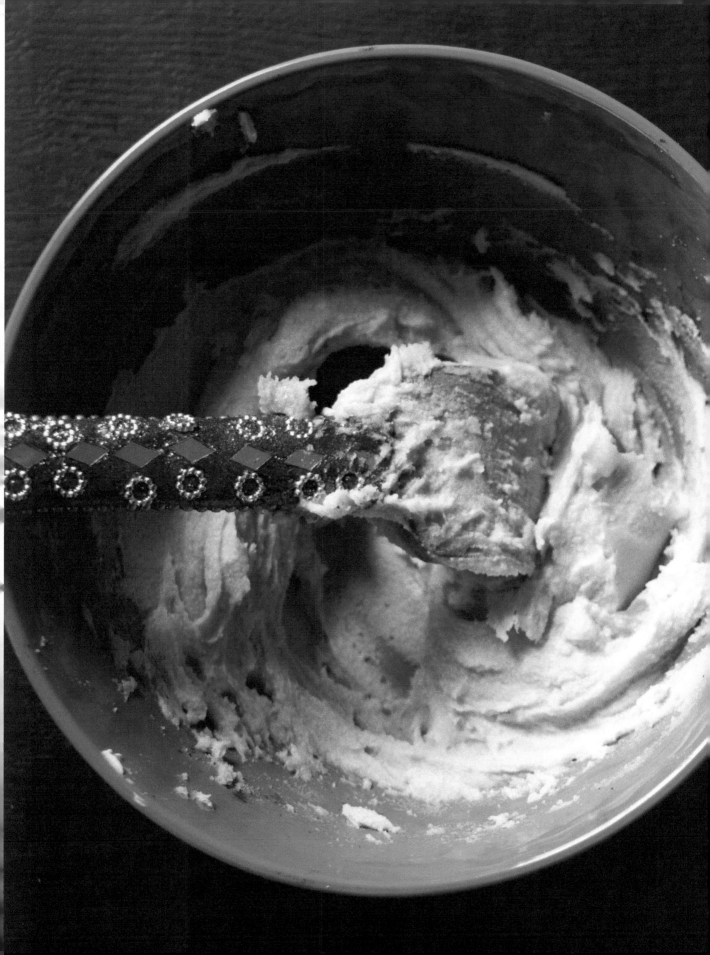

MAKE YOUR OWN BODY BUTTERS

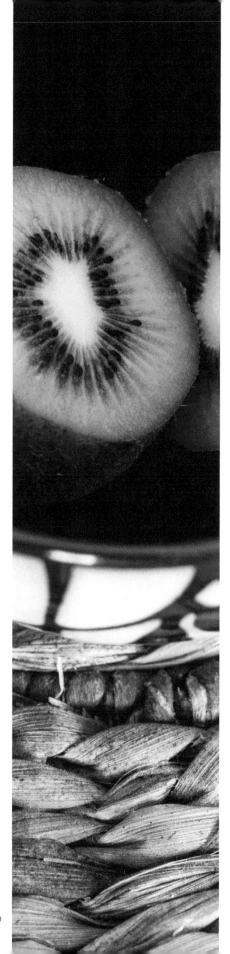

Kiwi Body Scrub

with
Sweet Almond Oil

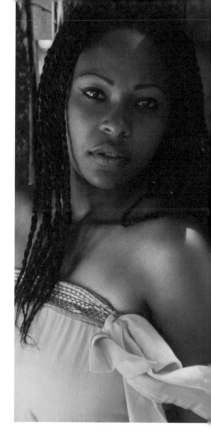

Kiwis 4, peeled and mashed
Plain yogurt 2 tbsp
Sweet Almond Oil 4 oz
Your favorite essential oil* 4 drops

1. Mix all ingredients, until smooth. Apply to skin as a scrub.

*Essential oils are highly potent and should be used with care. Follow all safety precautions from manufacturer when using essential oils. Please consult physician before extensive use of essential oils.

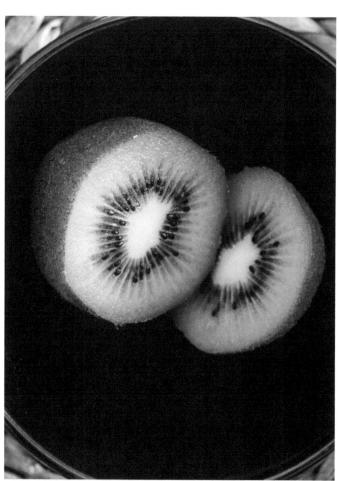

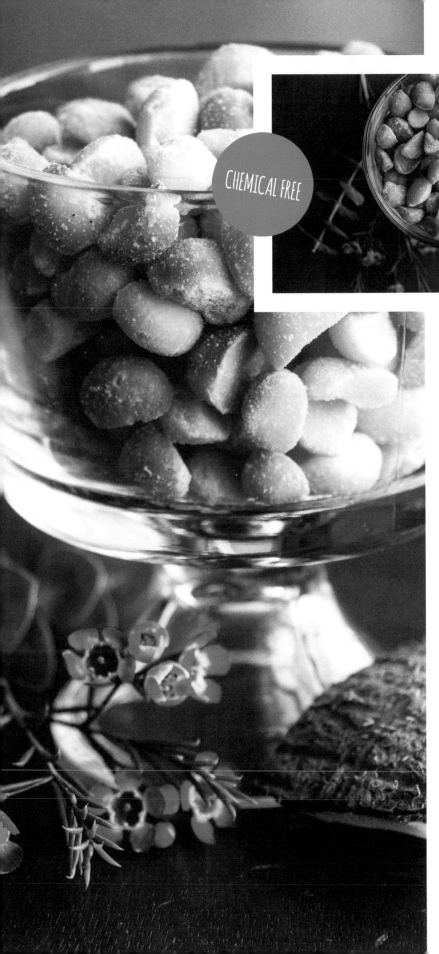

Macadamia Nut Body Butter

with
Coconut Oil

Macadamia Nut butter 4 ozs
Shea butter 4 ozs
Coconut oil 4 ozs
Sweet almond oil 4 ozs
Your favorite essential oil* 4 drops

1. In a stainless-steel saucepan, melt all the ingredients except the essential oil over low heat.
2. Remove from heat and keep stirring.
3. In a stainless-steel saucepan, melt all the ingredients except the essential oil over low heat.
4. When the mixture gets to room temperature, stir in the essential oils and continue stirring until smooth. Use a hand-mixer if necessary.

*Essential oils are highly potent and should be used with care. Follow all safety precautions from manufacturer when using essential oils. Please consult physician before extensive use of essential oils.

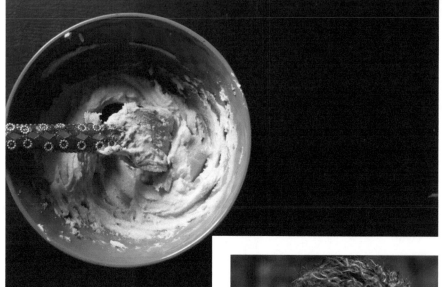

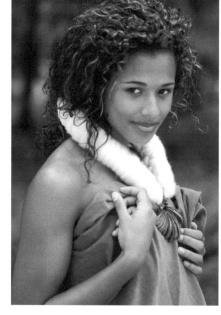

THE BENEFITS OF CHOCOLATE

Cacao is known for delighting the taste buds of lovers of all things sweet for centuries! What is relatively unknown is its benefits in skin care.

Cocoa butter is more widely known for its moisturizing and healing properties but when you add the chocolate extract to the mix you are introducing a highly beneficial spectrum of skin loving minerals including magnesium. For an added benefit, you get to enjoy the aromatherapy of delicious chocolate as you slather on this body butter!

ENJOY THE AROMATHERAPY OF DELICIOUS CHOCOLATE!

Chocolate Almond Body Butter

Cocoa butter ½ oz
Sweet almond oil 2 tbsp
Coconut oil 2 ozs
Beeswax ½ oz
Mineral water 2 ozs
Lemongrass essential oil* 1 tsp
Chocolate (Cacao) extract 2 drops
Peppermint essential oil* ½ tsp

1. In a stainless-steel saucepan, melt the beeswax and cocoa butter with the coconut oil over low heat.
2. Mix in the mineral water with a wooden spoon.
3. Remove from heat and keep stirring.
4. When the mixture gets to room temperature, stir in the essential oils and extract until mixture is smooth.
5. Keep shaking cream until the mixture is cooled completely as this will ensure that the oil and water do not separate.
6. Use a dark jar or store jar in a dark place to protect the essential oils from light.

*Essential oils are highly potent and should be used with care. Follow all safety precautions from manufacturer when using essential oils. Please consult physician before extensive use of essential oils.

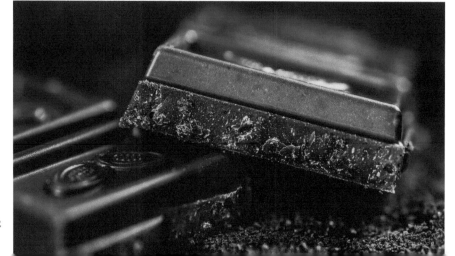

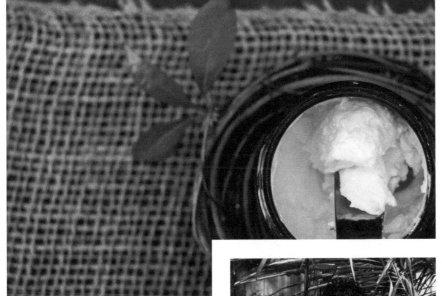

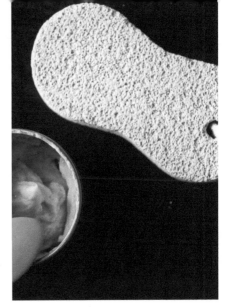

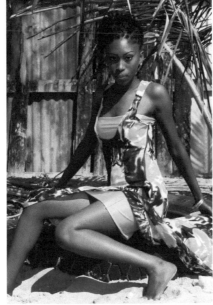

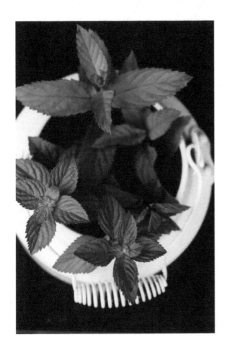

Peppermint Foot Cream

Coconut oil 2 oz
Calendula oil 1 oz
Beeswax ½ oz
Shea butter ½ oz
Mineral water 2 ½ oz
Peppermint essential oil* 1 tsp
Tea tree oil* ¼ tsp

1. In a stainless-steel saucepan, melt the Shea butter and beeswax with the Coconut and Calendula oils over low heat.
2. Mix in the mineral water with a wooden spoon.
3. Remove from heat and keep stirring.
4. When the mixture gets to room temperature, stir in the essential oils until mixture is smooth.
5. Keep stirring cream until the mixture is cooled completely. This will ensure that the oil and water do not separate.
6. Use a dark jar or store jar in a dark place to protect the essential oils from light.

*Essential oils are highly potent and should be used with care. Follow all safety precautions from manufacturer when using essential oils. Please consult physician before extensive use of essential oils.

BLAST FROM THE PAST BEST SELLER!

A blast from the past! This was a number one seller in the Janelle Beauty lineup back in the day. The cool, refreshing aroma of the peppermint was enough to put a bounce in your step!

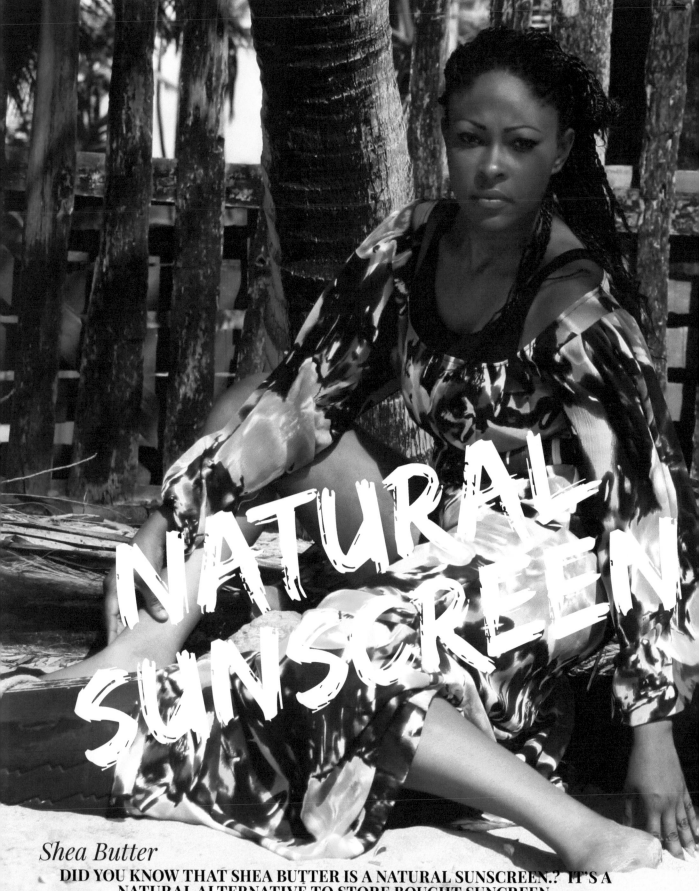

NATURAL SUNSCREEN

Shea Butter
DID YOU KNOW THAT SHEA BUTTER IS A NATURAL SUNSCREEN.? IT'S A NATURAL ALTERNATIVE TO STORE BOUGHT SUNCREEN.

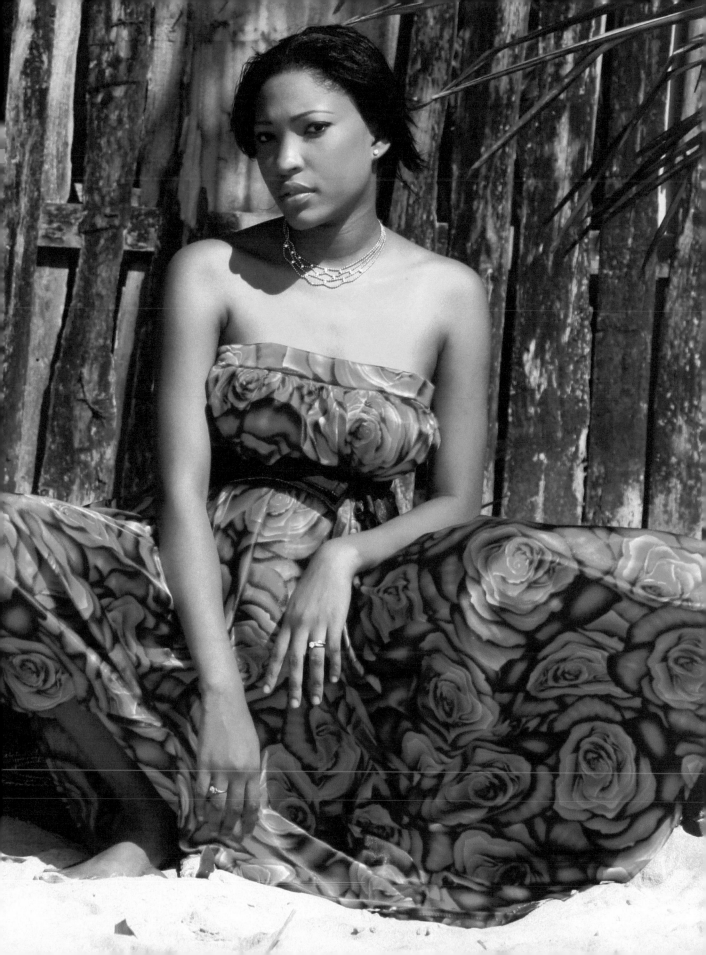

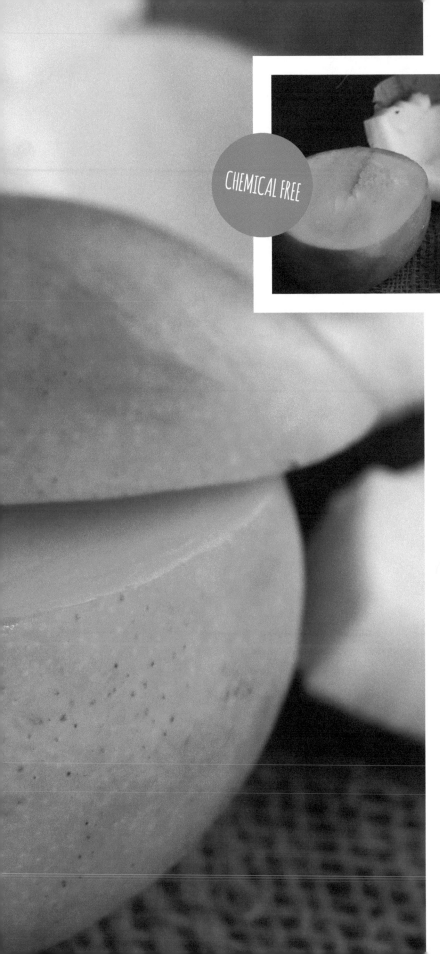

Mango Body Butter

with
Jojoba Oil

Mango butter 4 oz
Jojoba oil 4 oz
Your favorite essential oil* 4 drops

1. In a stainless-steel saucepan, melt all the ingredients except the essential oil over low heat.
2. Remove from heat and keep stirring.
3. When the mixture gets to room temperature, stir in the essential oils until mixture is smooth. Use a hand mixture if necessary.

*Essential oils are highly potent and should be used with care. Follow all safety precautions from manufacturer when using essential oils. Please consult physician before extensive use of essential oils.

janelle

Coco
body pol

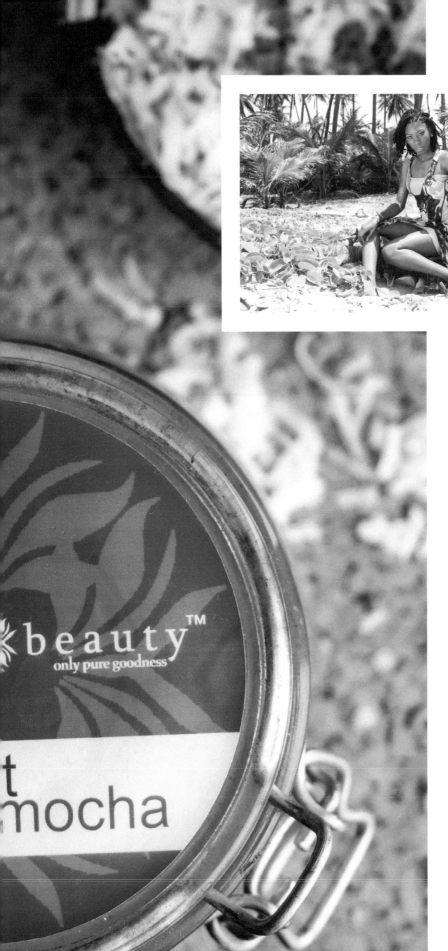

Coconut Mocha Body Polish

Whoever knew coffee beans can be a prized cosmetic ingredient? Coffee is beyond rich in anti-oxidants and its caffeine content draws out extra moisture and tightens skin. The grinds itself acts as an exfoliant that polishes away dead skin.

Ground coffee 9 ozs
Coconut oil 1 oz
Jojoba oil 4 ozs
Rosehip oil 1 tsp
German chamomile essential oil* 3 drops
Lime essential oil* 1 drop
Chocolate extract 2 drops

1. Combine all the ingredients into bowl and stir well. heat and keep stirring.

*Essential oils are highly potent and should be used with care. Follow all safety precautions from manufacturer when using essential oils. Please consult physician before extensive use of essential oils.

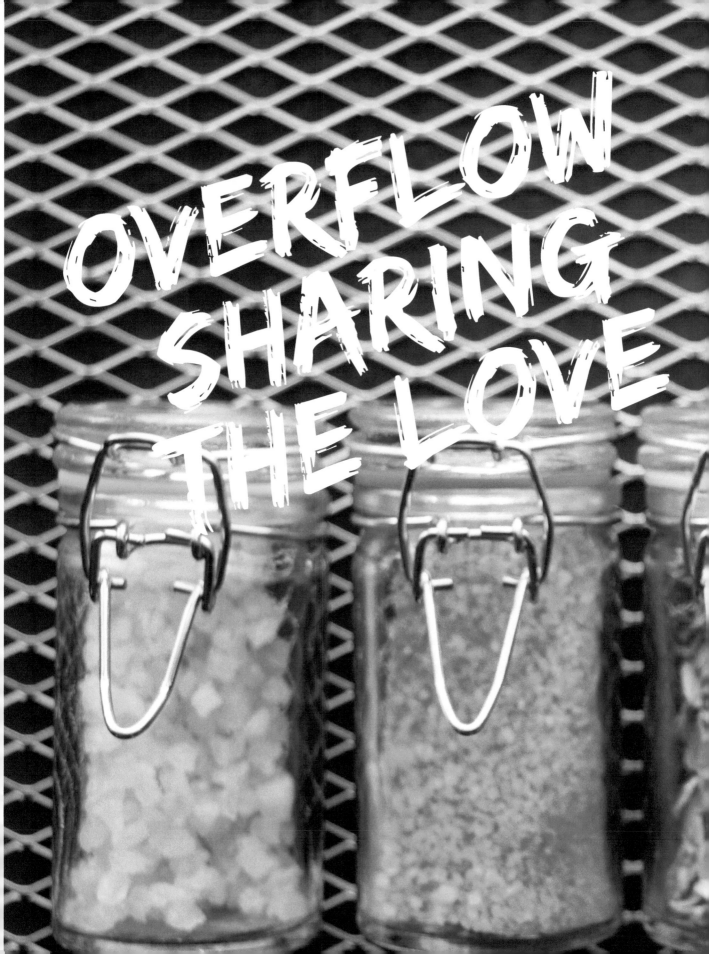

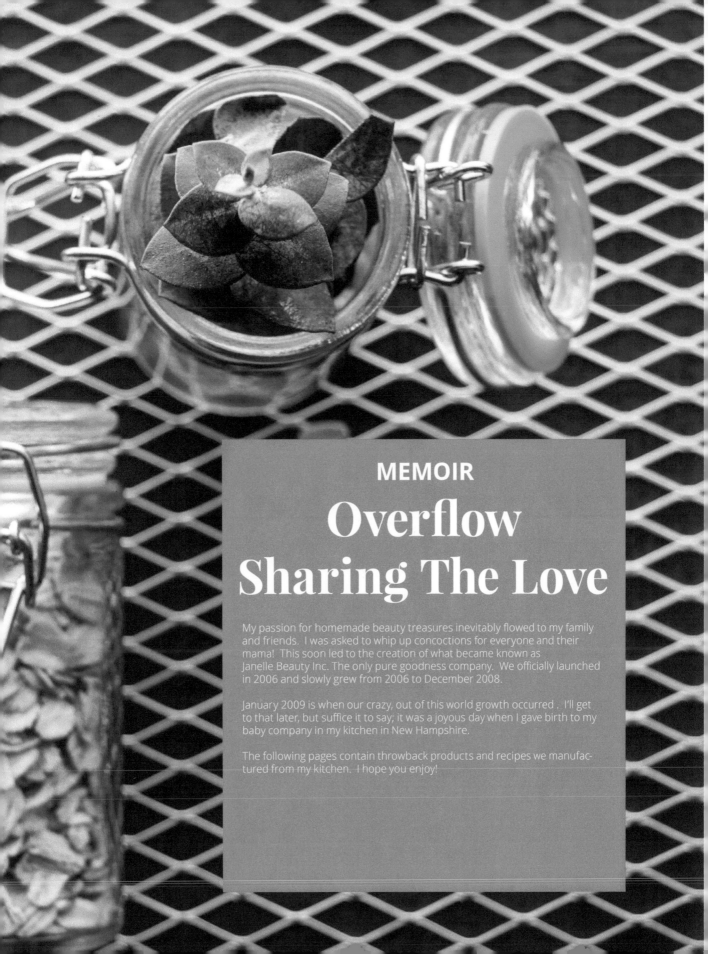

MEMOIR

Overflow
Sharing The Love

My passion for homemade beauty treasures inevitably flowed to my family and friends. I was asked to whip up concoctions for everyone and their mama! This soon led to the creation of what became known as Janelle Beauty Inc. The only pure goodness company. We officially launched in 2006 and slowly grew from 2006 to December 2008.

January 2009 is when our crazy, out of this world growth occurred . I'll get to that later, but suffice it to say; it was a joyous day when I gave birth to my baby company in my kitchen in New Hampshire.

The following pages contain throwback products and recipes we manufactured from my kitchen. I hope you enjoy!

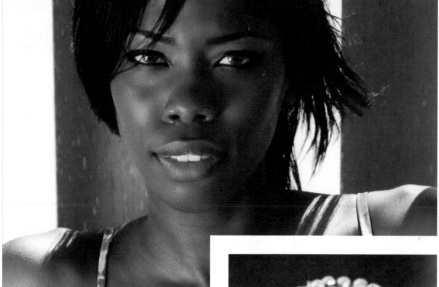

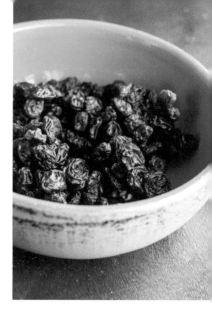

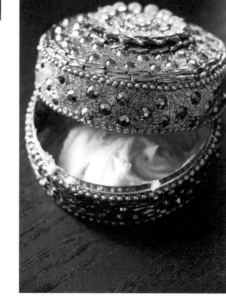

THE BENEFITS OF GRAPESEED

Don't throw out those pesky grapeseeds! With the proliferation of seedless grapes, we may soon have a generation that are not aware that grapeseeds even exist!

Grapeseeds give us the beauty treasure grapeseed oil which is rich in anti-oxidant, inflammatory properties and healthy fats. It is a prized beauty ingredient with a complex vitamin spectrum that moisturizes and tightens loose skin. It is light and easily absorbed and acts as a balance against oily skin.

Grapeseed Facial Cream

Grapeseed oil 1 1/2 fl oz
Jojoba oil 1 fl oz
Beeswax 1/2 oz
Mineral water 2 tbsp
Ylang-ylang essential oil* 2 drops
Calendula essential oil* 1 drop

1. In a stainless-steel pan, melt the oils (Grapeseed and Jojoba) and beeswax.
2. Slightly heat the mineral water and bea it slowly into the mixture.
3. Remove from heat and continuously sti until the cream gets to room temperature
4. Mix in the essential oils and combine until texture is smooth.
5. Spoon the cream into a glass jar and cover with lid.
6. Keep shaking cream until the mixture is cooled completely as this will ensure that the oil and water do not separate.
7. Use a dark jar or store jar in a dark plac to protect the essential oils from light.

*Essential oils are highly potent and shoul be used with care. Follow all safety precau tions from manufacturer when using essen tial oils. Please consult physician before extensive use of essential oils.

EXCELLENT FOR OILY SKIN

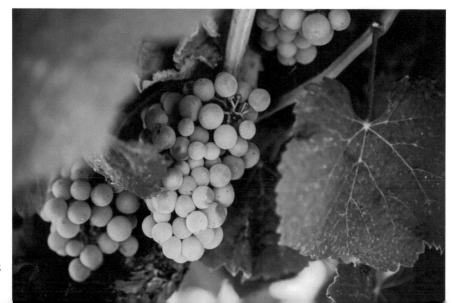

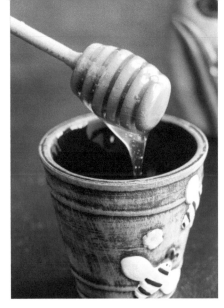

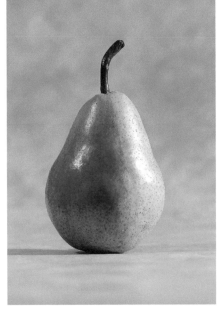

THE BENEFITS OF PEAR

The nutrient dense pear is full of hydroxy-cinnamic acids and flavonoids, both of which renders its skin nurturing effects when ingested and applied topically.

The pear itself acts as a gentle exfoliant by removing dead skin which in turn allows the nutrients in the mashed pears to be delivered to the skin.

Pears are also rich in anti-oxidants and vita-min C which is known to aid in the reduction of the appearance of wrinkles.

Pear & Honey Facial Mask

1 Pear peeled and chopped in small pieces
Raw honey 1/2 tsp
Yogurt 1 tsp

1. Mix ingredients in a bowl with a fork, mashing the pear into the honey and yogurt.
2. Let infuse for an hour.
3. Apply mask to skin with fingers.
4. Rinse after 15 minutes with cool water.

LACTIC ACID IN YOGURT IS GREAT FOR TIGHTENING SKIN

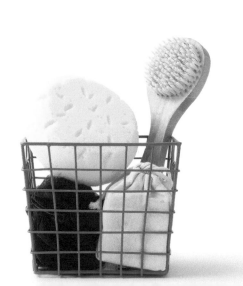

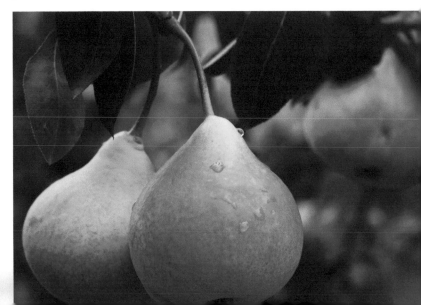

TONING
facial rinse

Oh the wonders of the super-ingredient Apple Cider Vinegar! It is simply a powerhouse that don't need a lot of support from other ingredients to shine.

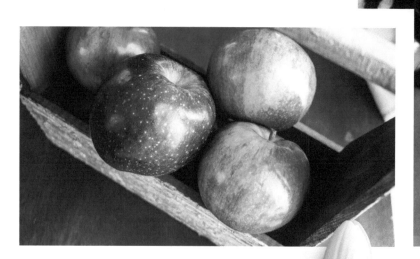

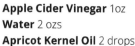

Apple Cider Vinegar 1oz
Water 2 ozs
Apricot Kernel Oil 2 drops

1. Mix Apple Cider Vinegar and water in a glass bowl.
2. Apply with cotton ball to skin to tone and clean skin. Pat dry.
3. Apply Apricot Kernel Oil to moisturize.

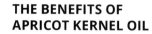

THE BENEFITS OF APRICOT KERNEL OIL

The precious seeds of Apricots are bursting with nutrients and is anti-everything bad! It is anti–inflammatory, anti-aging, anti–bacterial, anti-septic and an anti-oxidant.

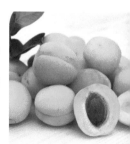

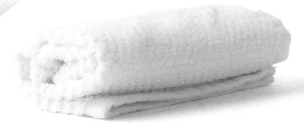

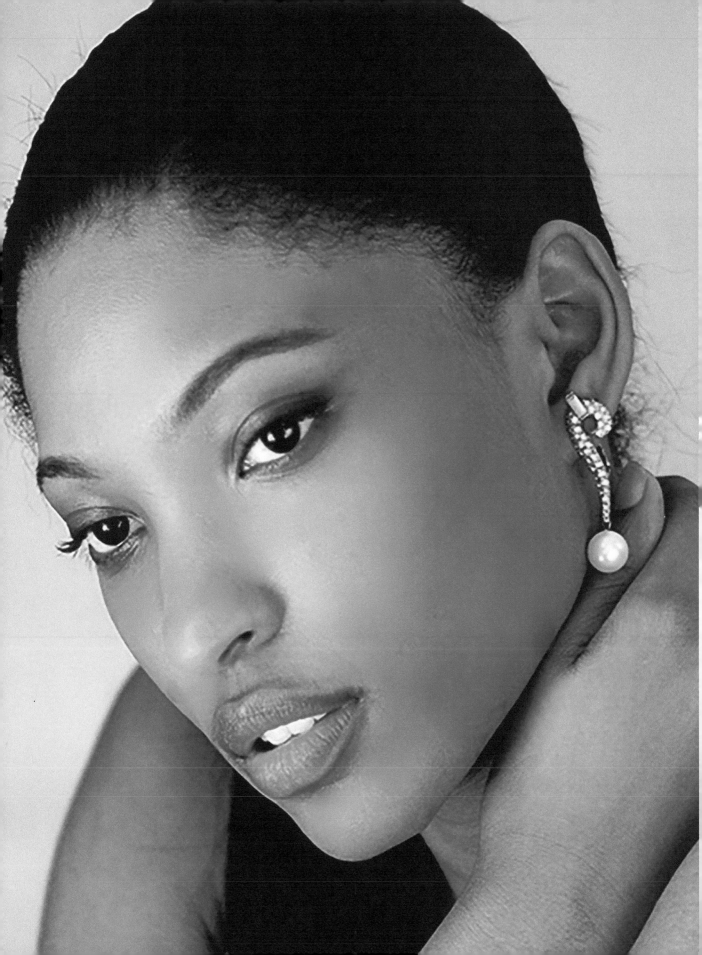

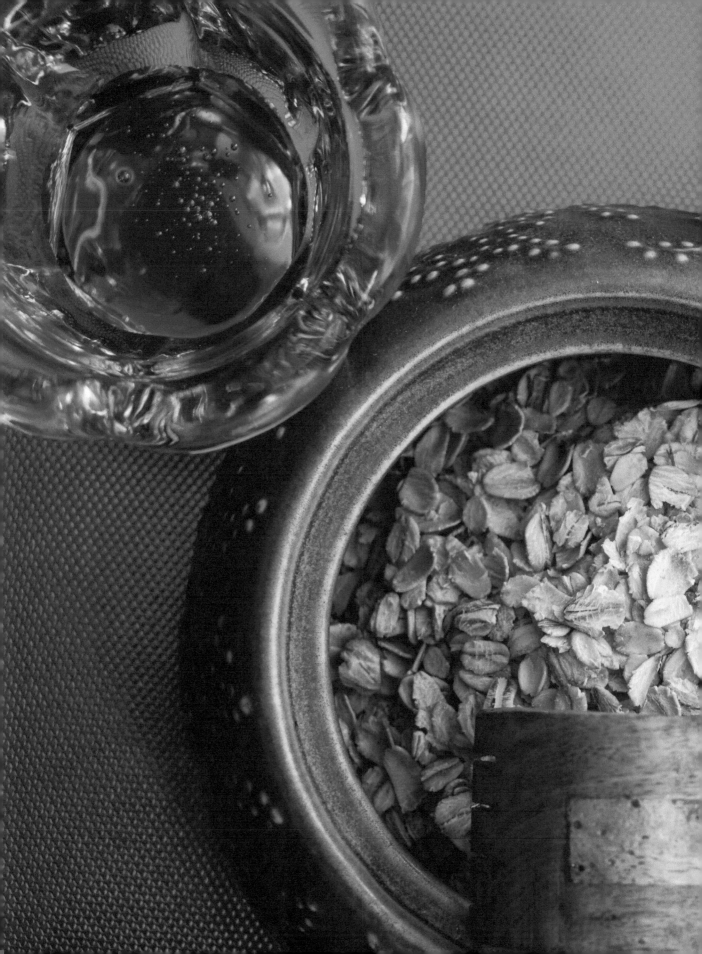

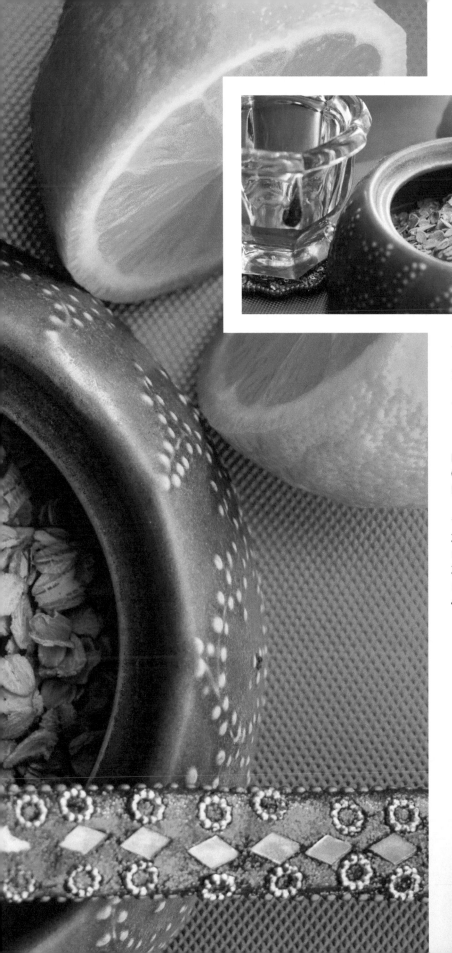

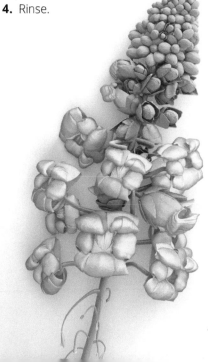

Honey & Oats Facial Scrub

Honey 2 tbsp
Oats 1 cup
Lemon juice 1 tsp

1. Mix all ingredients in a glass bowl.
2. Apply to skin with gentle scrubbing motions.
3. May leave on as a mask for 10 minutes.
4. Rinse.

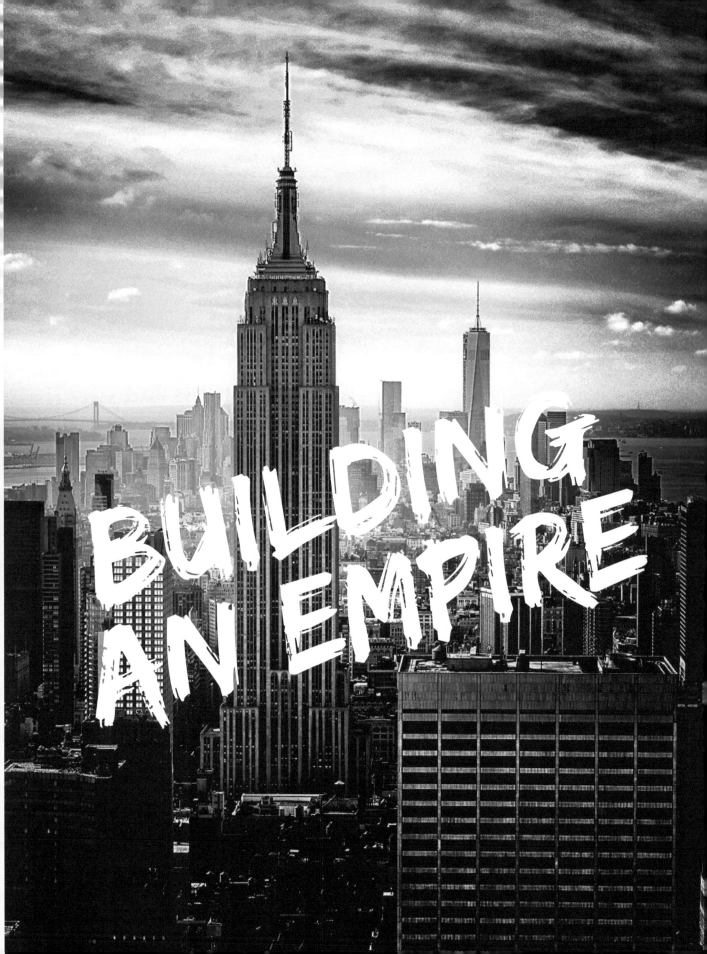

PRIDE: Building an Empire

We were growing so fast that we could not keep up.

It got to the point where demand outpaced supply and our operating structure was struggling to keep up.

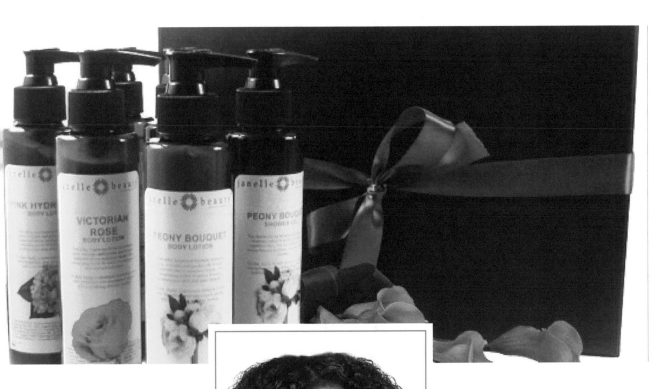

As we grew as a company, one thing led to another, and I was approached by many companies and people with their own products who wanted to partner with my growing baby, Janelle Beauty.

We took on a product that was in its infancy and nurtured it under the growing Janelle Beauty umbrella. We reinvested our resources to keep up with marketing costs and it paid off.

It was a huge success! We were growing so fast that we could not keep up. It got to the point where **demand outpaced supply** and our operating structure was struggling to keep up.

What happened as a result was not pretty; however, we kept making products as we tottered on the brink of disaster. I was not interested in outside investment or loans so we were on our own.

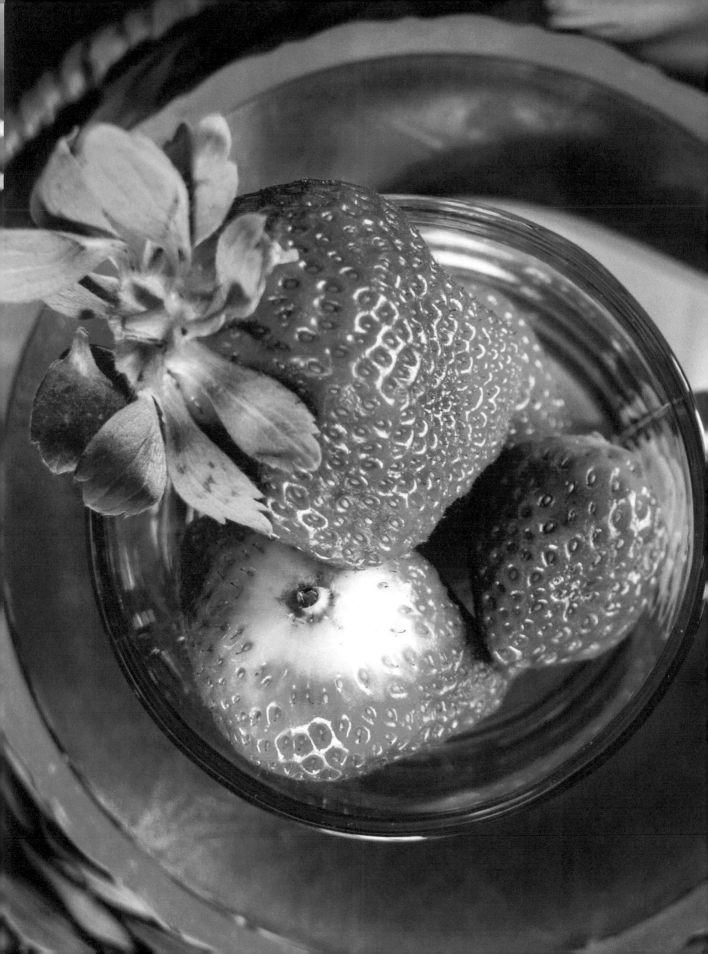

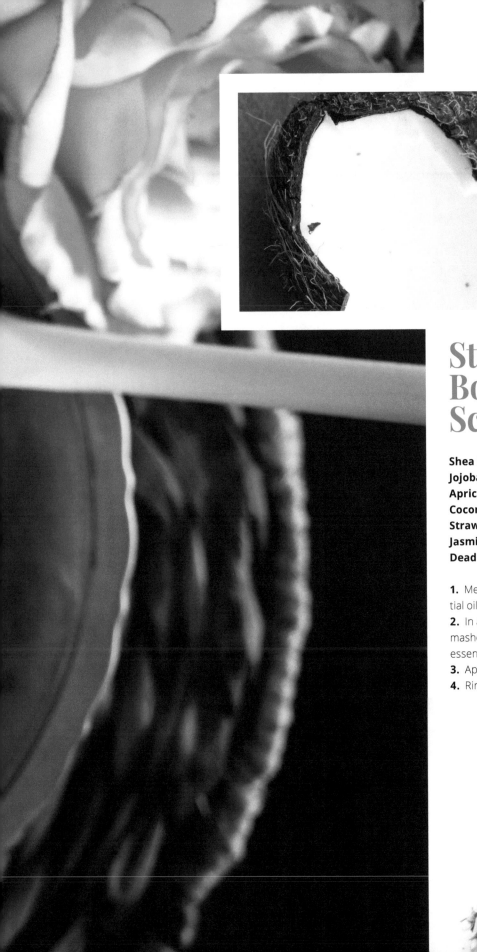

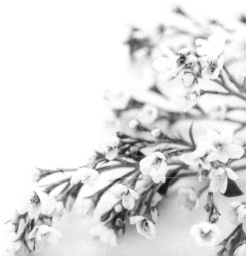

Strawberry Body Butter-Scrub

Shea Butter 2 ozs
Jojoba Oil 1 tsp
Apricot Oil 1 tsp
Coconut Oil 1 oz
Strawberries 1 cup
Jasmine essential oil 2 drops
Dead Sea Salt 1 cup

1. Melt shea butter with oils except essential oil.
2. In a bowl, combine melted mixture with mashed strawberries, Dead Sea salt and essential oil.
3. Apply to skin with scrubbing motions.
4. Rinse and pat dry.

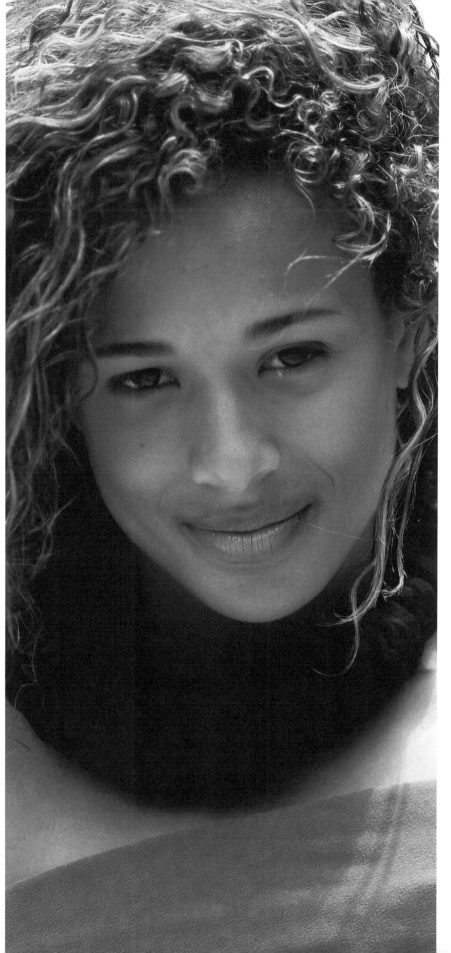

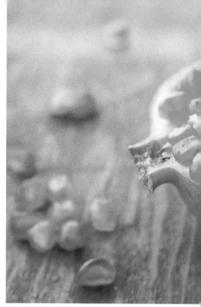

Pomegranate Facial Cream

Wheatgerm oil 1 1/2 fl oz
Pomegranate oil 1 fl oz
Beeswax 1/2 oz
Mineral water 2 tbsp
Rose essential oil* 2 drops
Patchouli essential oil* 1 drop

1. In a stainless-steel pan, melt the oils (Wheatgerm and Pomegranate) and bees wax.
2. Slightly heat the mineral water and be it slowly into the mixture.
3. Remove from heat and continuously s until the cream gets to room temperatur
4. Mix in the essential oils and combine until texture is smooth.
5. Spoon the cream into a glass jar and cover with lid.
6. Keep shaking cream until the mixture i cooled completely as this will ensure that the oil and water do not separate.
7. Use a dark jar or store jar in a dark plac to protect the essential oils from light.

*Essential oils are highly potent and shou be used with care. Follow all safety precau tions from manufacturer when using esse tial oils. Please consult physician before extensive use of essential oils.

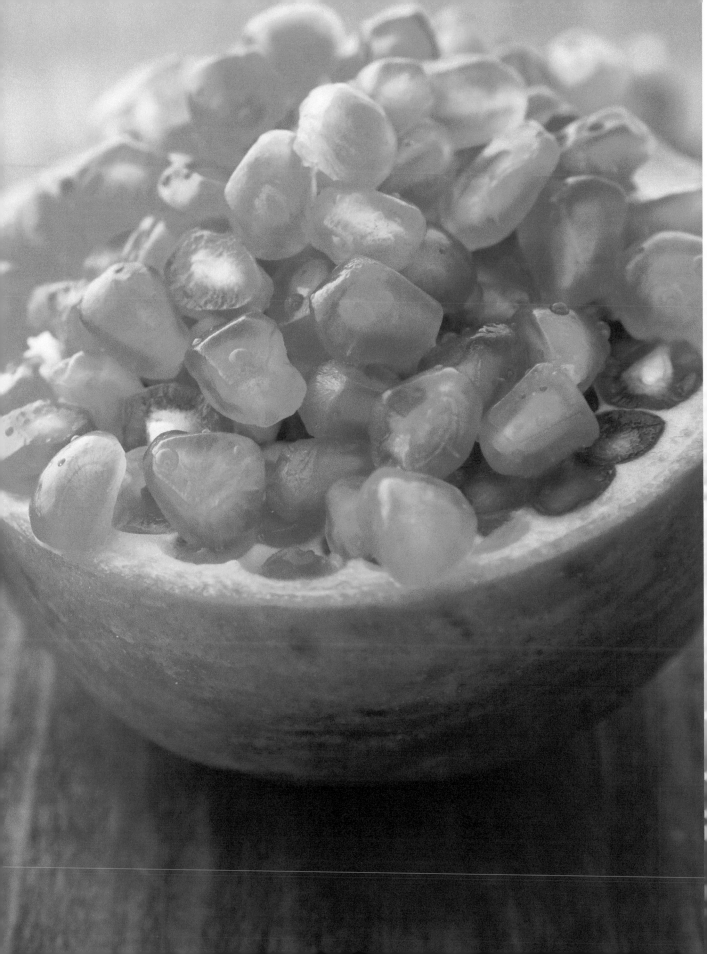

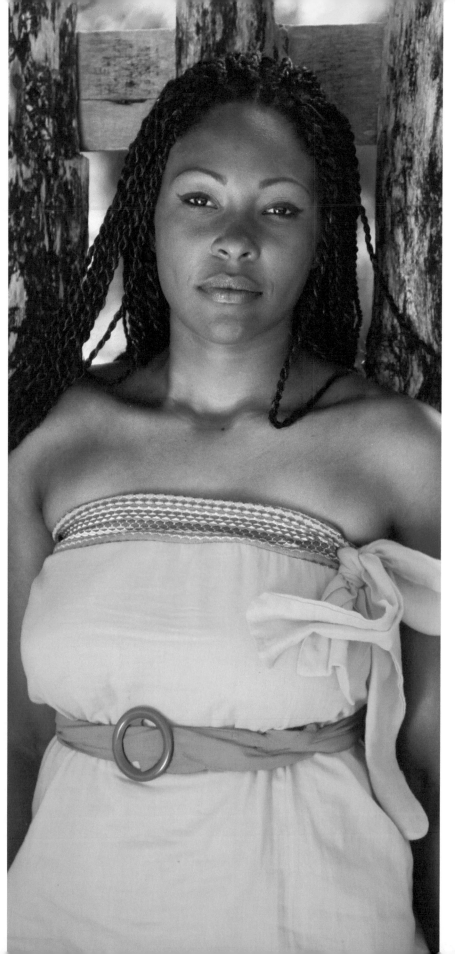

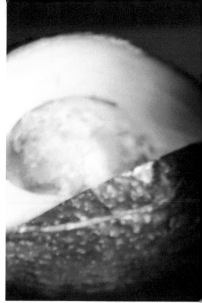

Avocado
Facial Cream

Olive oil 1 1/2 fl oz
Avocado oil 1 fl oz
Beeswax 1/2 oz
Mineral water 2 tbsp
Rosemary essential oil* 2 drops
Neroli essential oil* 1 drop

1. In a stainless-steel pan, melt the oils (Olive and Avocado) and beeswax.
2. Slightly heat the mineral water and bea it slowly into the mixture.
3. Remove from heat and continuously st until the cream gets to room temperature
4. Mix in the essential oils and combine until texture is smooth.
5. Spoon the cream into a glass jar and cover with lid.
6. Keep shaking cream until the mixture i cooled completely as this will ensure that the oil and water do not separate.
7. Use a dark jar or store jar in a dark plac to protect the essential oils from light.

*Essential oils are highly potent and shoul be used with care. Follow all safety precau tions from manufacturer when using esse tial oils. Please consult physician before extensive use of essential oils.

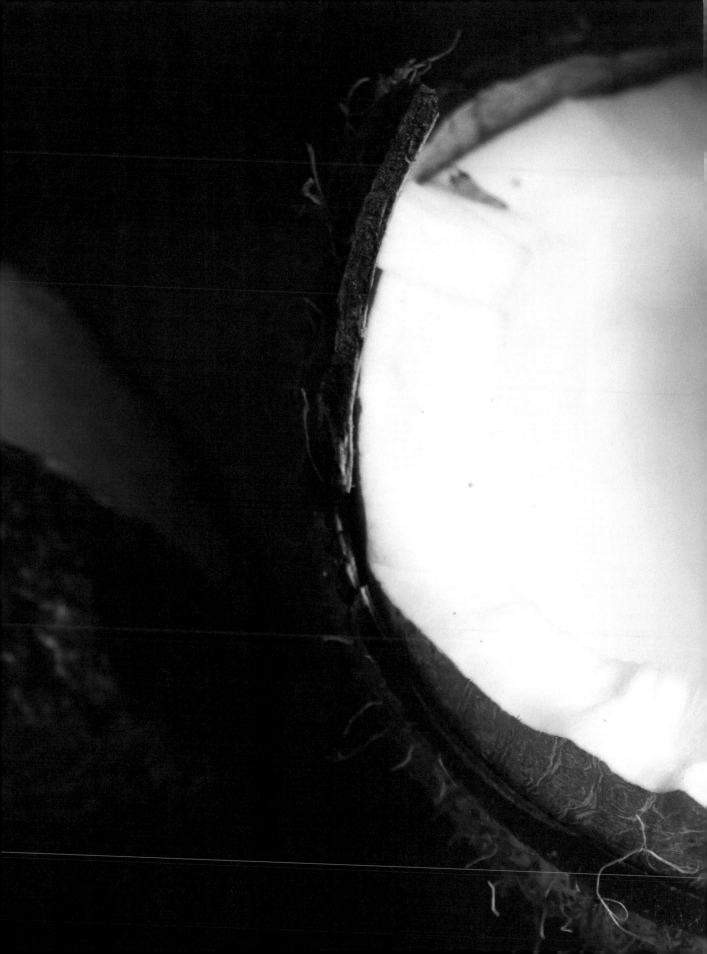

DESTRUCTION
Death of a Vision

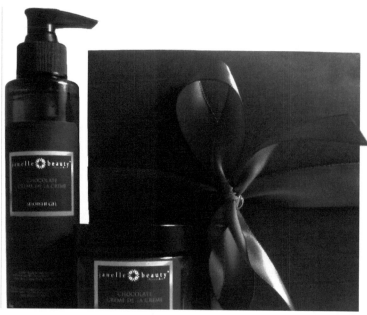

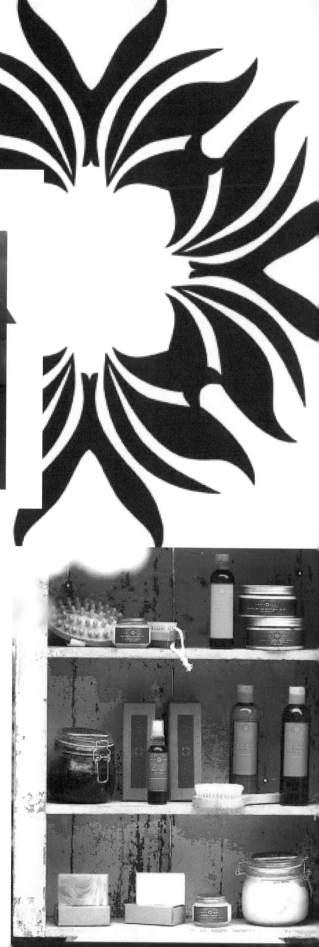

Well it finally happened. Our burn rate, got to the point of ashes. We had too many orders to keep up with and too many expenses to cover and not enough capital to keep inventory on hand. Customers were waiting months for their products and any goodwill we had built up with our customers were beginning to fizzle out.

I was at an impasse with the management team and we did not have the same priorities on how to handle our mounting crisis. I take full responsibility for not taking the reins of the company and leading it the way I knew was right in my own eyes. As a result, when

I did take back control of my company, I decided to shut down all retail sales until we could catch up with our backorders.

It was a devastating time for me.

A lot of people were congratulating me on having **the best problem in the world - too many orders;** but I knew the heartache of not taking control when I should of and not fighting harder to endure the growth phase.

Inevitably, my vision for my toddler company died.

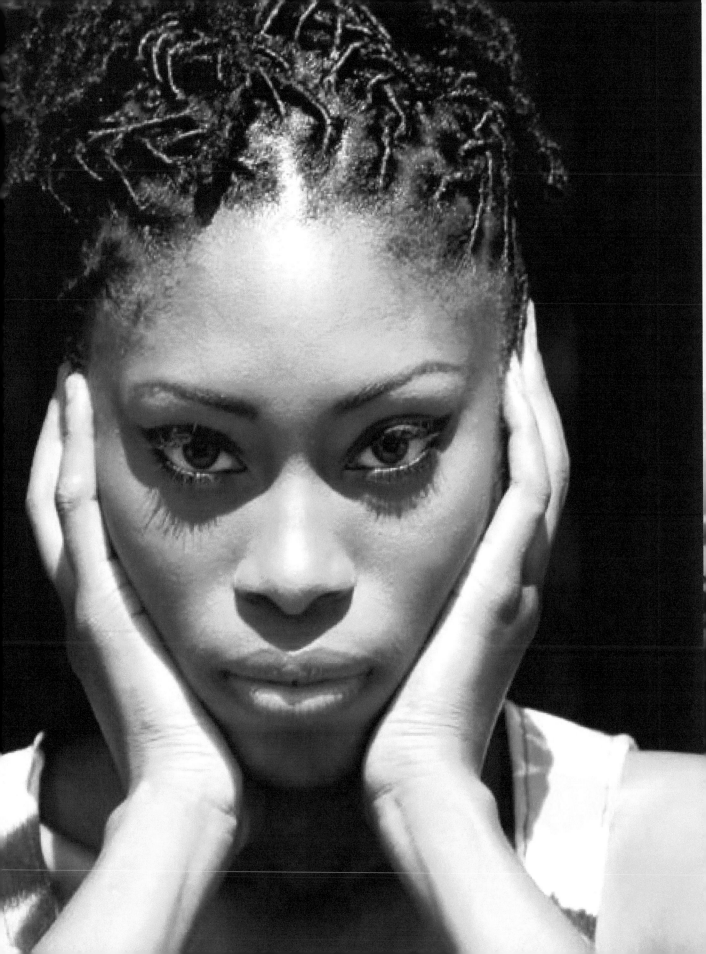

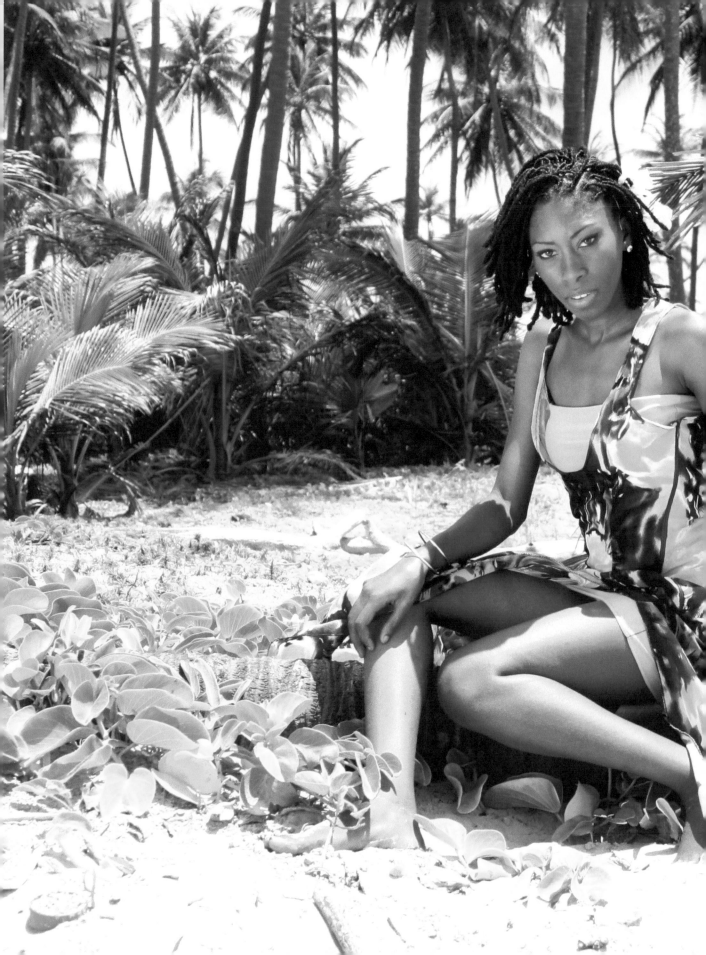

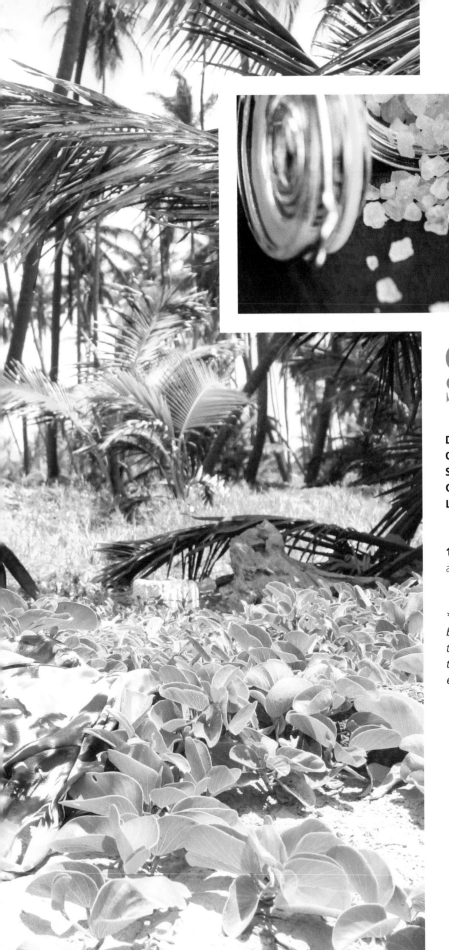

Ginger Bath Salts

Dead Sea Salt 4 ozs
Coconut oil 1 tsp
Sweet almond oil 1 tsp
Ginger essential oil* 3 drops
Lemongrass essential oil* 6 drops

1. Combine all the ingredients into bowl and stir well.

Essential oils are highly potent and should be used with care. Follow all safety precautions from manufacturer when using essential oils. Please consult physician before extensive use of essential oils.

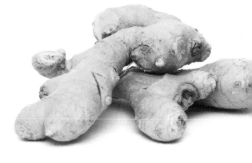

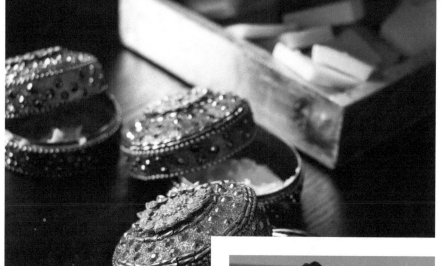

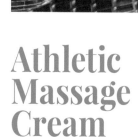

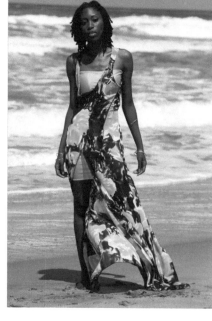

This massage cream contains the potent black pepper essential oil. This oil has a spicy and warm aroma that is both stimulating and empowering. Combined with rosemary, the fatigue-busting herb, this massage cream will alleviate muscle pain as you recover from the rigor of exercise.

Athletic Massage Cream

Coconut oil 2 ozs
Hazelnut oil 1 oz
Beeswax ½ oz
Shea Butter ½ oz
Mineral water 2 1/2 ozs
Rosemary essential oil* 1 ½ tsp
Black pepper essential oil* ½ tsp

1. In a stainless-steel pan, melt the Shea butter and beeswax with the Coconut and Hazelnut oils over low heat.
2. Mix in the mineral water with a wooden spoon until mixture is smooth.
3. Remove from heat and keep stirring.
4. When the mixture gets to room temperature, stir in the essential oils.
5. Spoon the cream into a glass jar and cover with lid.
6. Keep shaking cream until the mixture is cooled completely as this will ensure that the oil and water do not separate.
7. Use a dark jar or store jar in a dark place to protect the essential oils from light.

Essential oils are highly potent and should be used with care. Follow all safety precautions from manufacturer when using essential oils. Please consult physician before extensive use of essential oils.

KEEP SHAKING CREAM UNTIL THE MIXTURE IS COOLED COMPLETELY.

CHOCOLATE ALMOND FOOT LOTION

Cocoa butter ½ oz
Sweet almond oil 2 tbsp
Coconut oil 2 ozs
Beeswax ½ oz
Mineral water 2 ozs
Lemongrass essential oil* 1 tsp
Chocolate extract 2 drops
Peppermint essential oil* ½ tsp

1. In a stainless-steel saucepan, melt the beeswax and cocoa butter with the coconut oil over low heat.
2. Mix in the mineral water with a wooden spoon until mixture is smooth.
3. Remove from heat and keep stirring.
4. When the mixture gets to room temperature, stir in the essential oils.
5. Spoon the cream into a glass jar and cover with lid.
6. Keep shaking cream until the mixture is cooled completely as this will ensure that the oil and water do not separate.
7. Use a dark jar or store jar in a dark place to protect the essential oils from light.

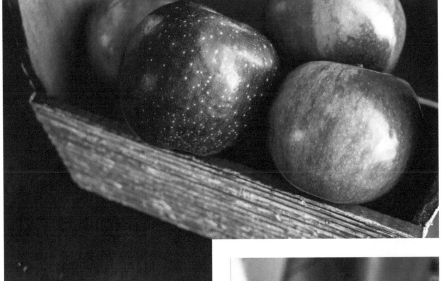

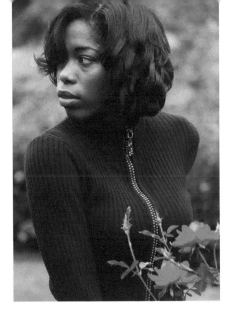

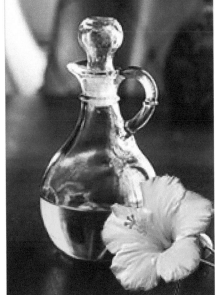

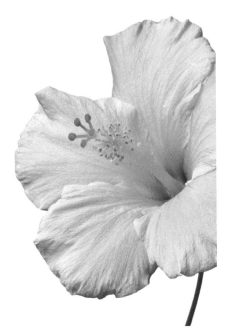

Hibiscus Hair Rinse

Hibiscus Tea 2 cups
Apple Cider Vinegar 1/2 cup
Filtered water 1 cup
Lavender essential oil* 10 drops

1. Combine all ingredients in a bowl.
2. Use right after shampooing. Rinse and continue your hair wash regimen. Shiny, bouncy hair awaits!

*Essential oils are highly potent and should be used with care. Follow all safety precautions from manufacturer when using essential oils. Please consult physician before extensive use of essential oils.

Shine Brighter Facial Cleanser

Lemon 1 tsp
Yogurt 1 tbsp
Lemon essential oil* 2 drops

1. Combine all the ingredients into bowl and stir well.

*Essential oils are highly potent and should be used with care. Follow all safety precautions from manufacturer when using essential oils. Please consult physician before extensive use of essential oils.

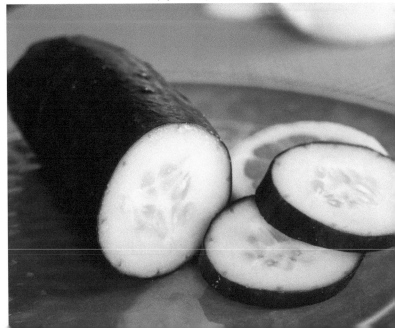

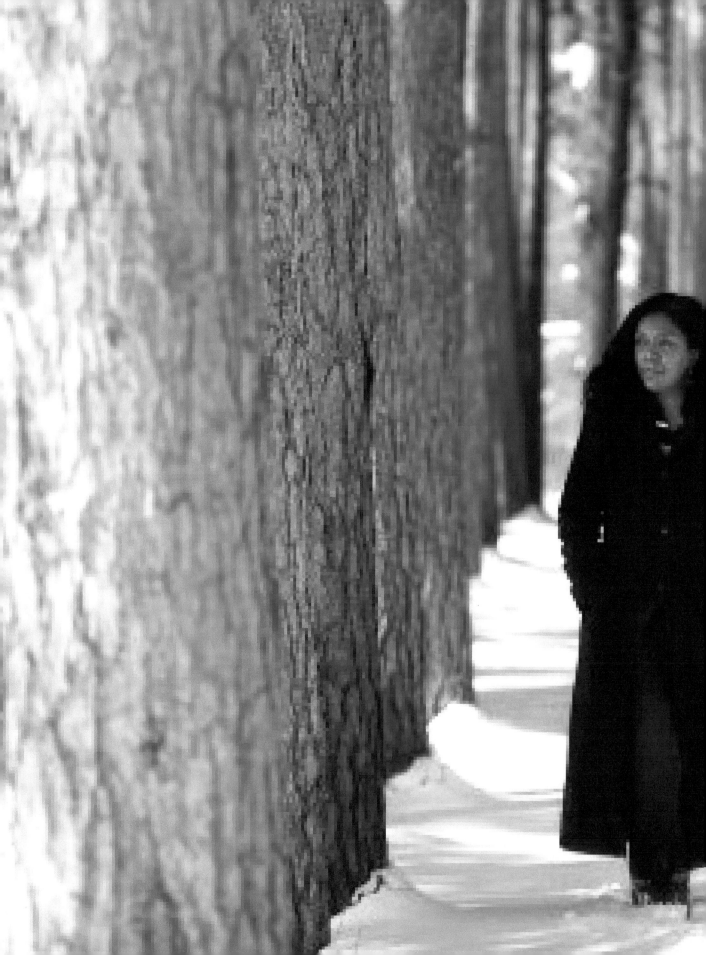

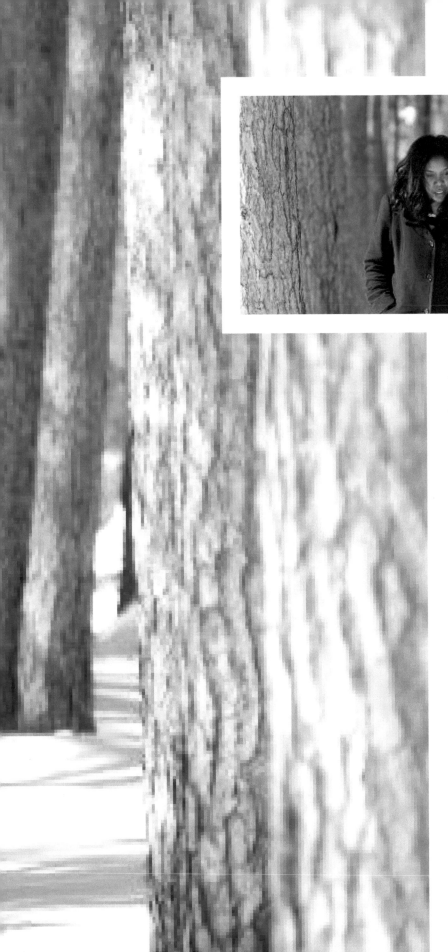

The Wilderness Years

During my time of hiatus, I started and co-founded several other companies. I buried myself in work helping others establish their brands and I fully utilized all the lessons learned in my Janelle Beauty endeavor to help others avoid the mistakes I made.

I was truly traumatized at what I considered a failure and a dead vision. However, I knew, deep down in my soul, that God was not done with Janelle Beauty yet. I had boldly declared as our company mantra in the early days that "In God we Trust."

I sincerely felt that I had let everyone down - my employees, my customers, my suppliers and most of all, my God. In the middle of all the new work I was involved with, I harbored a deep pain that no one but God could remove.

I knew the time would come when He would give me beauty for ashes.

It was just not my time yet.

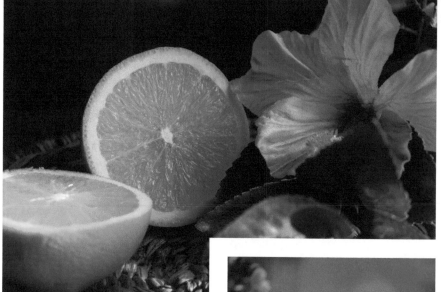

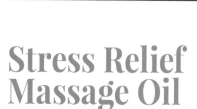

THE BENEFITS OF LAVENDER OIL

Many studies have been done on the effectiveness of lavender to combat anxiety, stress and even insomnia.

A single-blinded, randomized pilot study evaluating the aroma of Lavandula augustifolia as a treatment for mild insomnia resulted in favor of lavender.* Lavender has a long history of benefits and it has always been a prized treasure in beauty treatments.

* J Altern Complement Med 2005;11:631-7

Stress Relief Massage Oil

Sweet Almond Oil* 9 oz
Roman Chamomile essential oil** 5 drops
Mandarin essential oil 10 drops
Lavender essential oil 2 drops

1. Pour all ingredients in a dark glass bottle and shake gently.

2. Massage skin with oil as needed.

*If you are allergic to nuts, try substituting almond oil with sunflower oil

**Essential oils are highly potent and should be used with care. Follow all safety precautions from manufacturer when using essential oils. Please consult physician before extensive use of essential oils.

ELIMINATE STRESS WITH SOOTHING LAVENDER

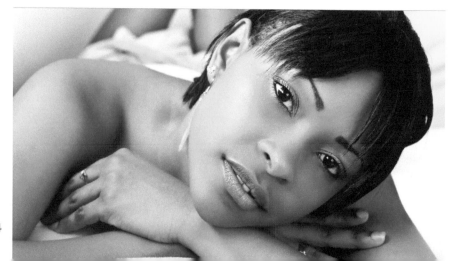

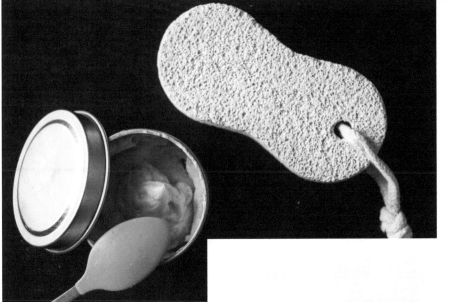

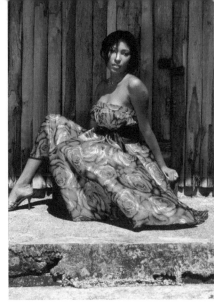

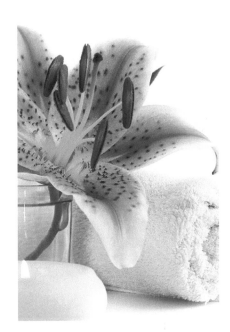

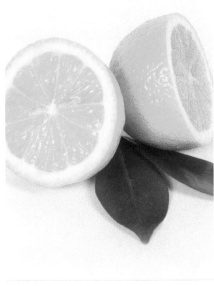

Pampered Cuticle Cream

Distilled water 5 ozs
Shea Butter 6 ozs
Glycerine 1.5 ozs
Lemon essential oil* 1/2 tsp
Young nettle tops 3 handfuls

1. Add nettle tops to boiling water and let boil for 10 minutes.
2. Melt shea butter in a saucepan over low heat.
3. Remove from heat and mix in the glycerine with a wooden spoon and slowly add the nettle mixture. Stir continuously.
4. When cream mixture is cooled to room temperature, add the essential oils.
5. Store in dark glass container to preserve the essential oils.

*Don't expose skin to sun when using citrus essential oils. Citrus essential oils make skin more sensitive to sunlight. Essential oils are highly potent and should be used with care. Follow all safety precautions from manufacturer when using essential oils. Please consult physician before extensive use of essential oils.

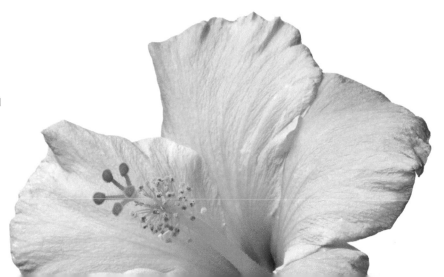

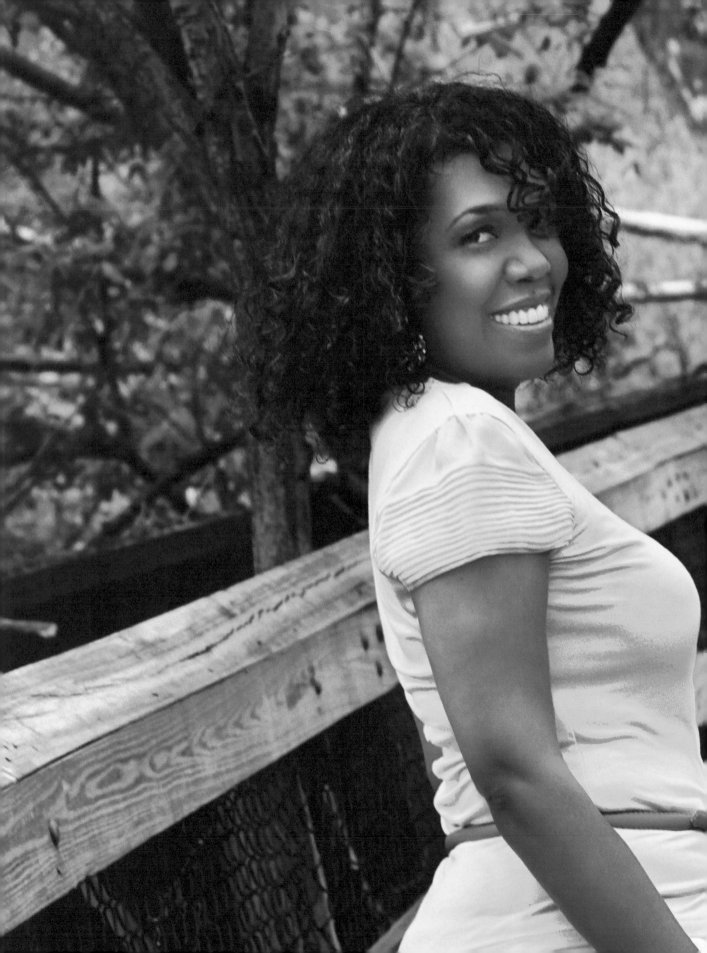

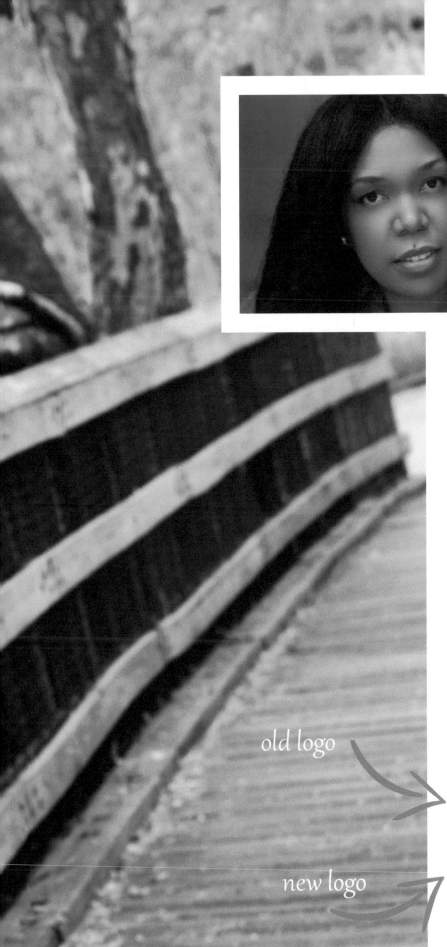

Resurrection: Greater Glory

God is good. He is faithful. One day, while minding the business of others (in a good way!) God finally called Janelle Beauty's name. In that moment, all the pain and regret and remorse vanished away and my vision was resurrected! I was free to pursue my dream again!

It was the most liberating moment of my life to date! This book was the first fruit of that resurrection. A simple memoir and a revealing of all the great homemade treasures that you can make on your own, as you pursue the "only pure goodness" lifestyle.

The first product I created back in 2005, Shine, will be made available again in mass production. Also, I am gearing up with a new team to produce the most amazing, only pure goodness, product line the world has ever seen!

old logo

janelle beauty™
only pure goodness

new logo

janelle beauty™
only pure goodness

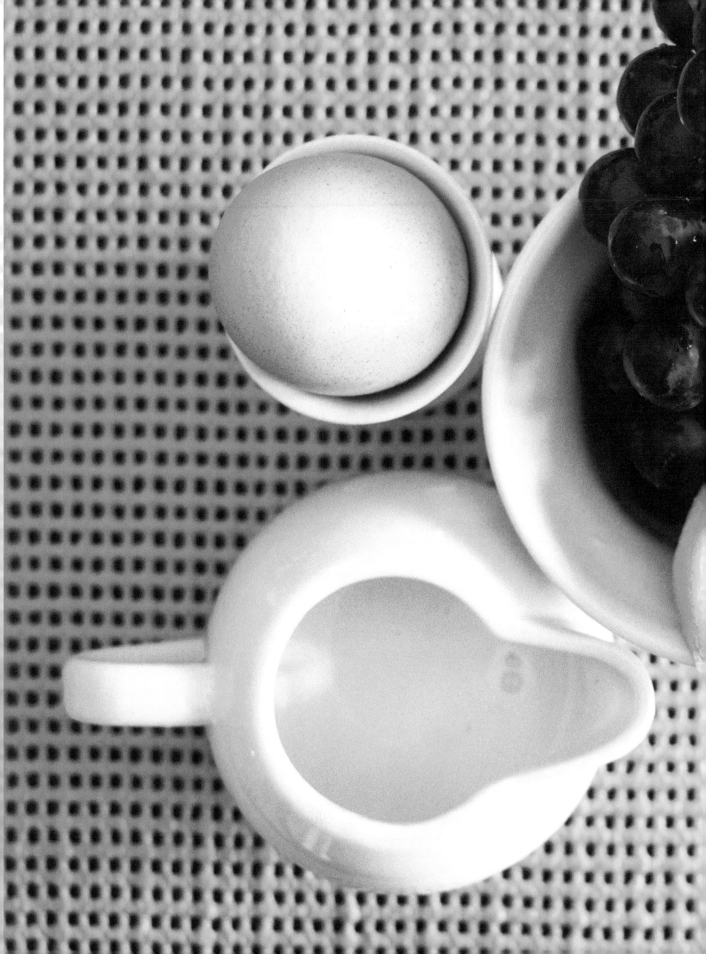

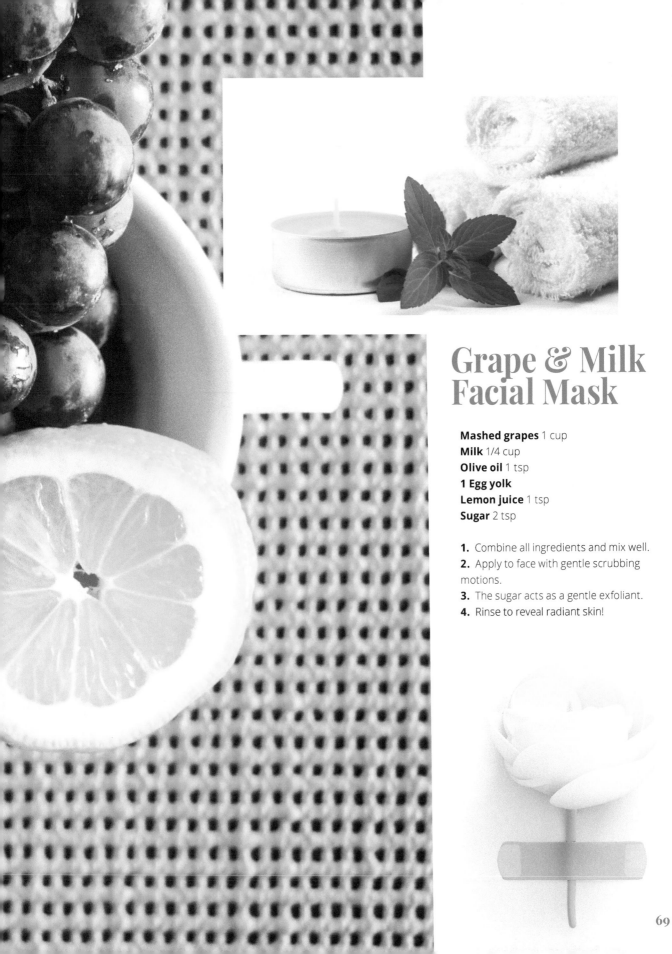

Grape & Milk Facial Mask

Mashed grapes 1 cup
Milk 1/4 cup
Olive oil 1 tsp
1 Egg yolk
Lemon juice 1 tsp
Sugar 2 tsp

1. Combine all ingredients and mix well.
2. Apply to face with gentle scrubbing motions.
3. The sugar acts as a gentle exfoliant.
4. Rinse to reveal radiant skin!

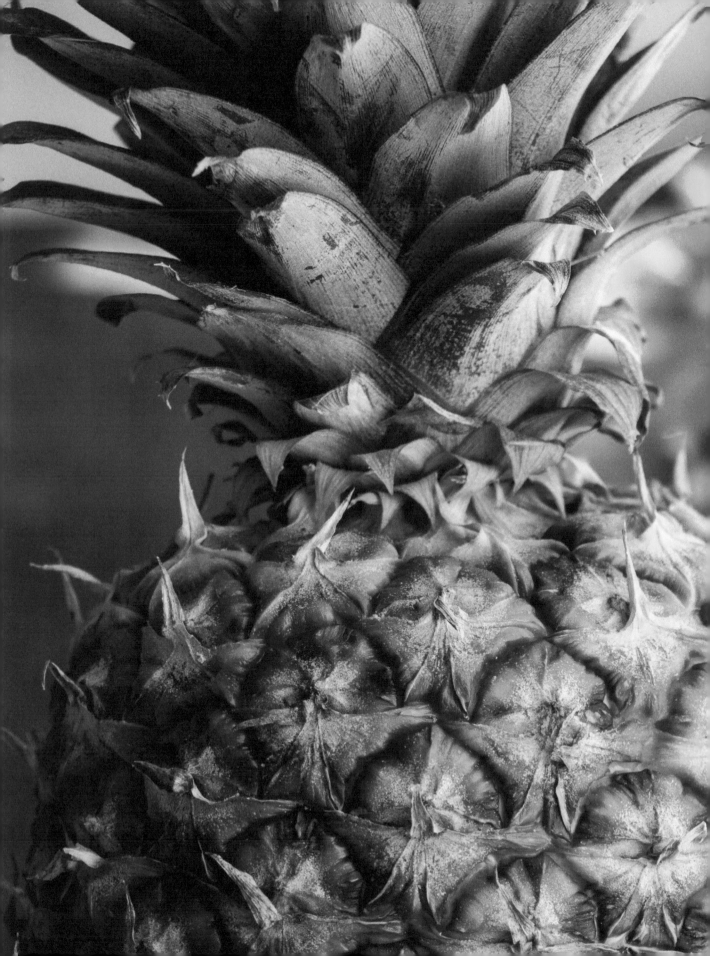

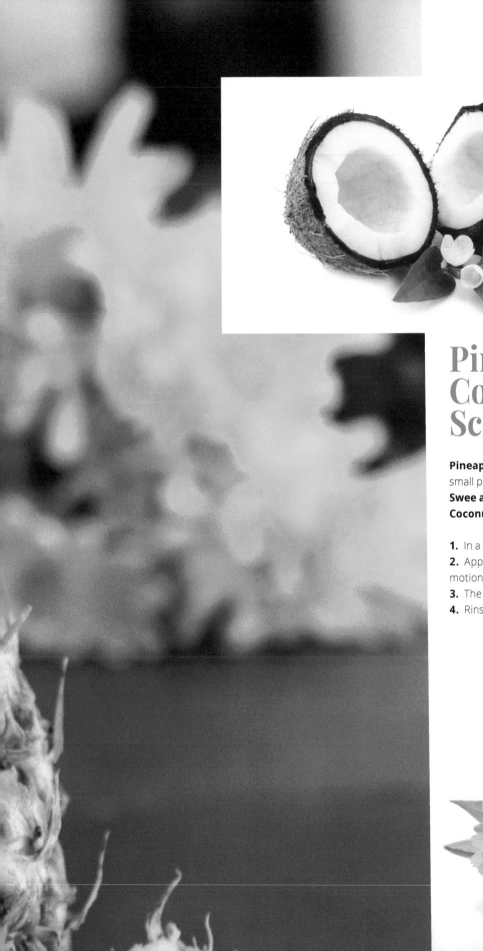

Pineapple Coconut Scrub

Pineapple 4 slices peeled and chopped in small pieces.
Swee almond oil 2 1/2 tsp
Coconut oil 2 tbsp

1. In a blender mix all ingredients
2. Apply to body with gentle scrubbing motions.
3. The pineapple acts as a gentle exfoliant.
4. Rinse to reveal radiant skin!

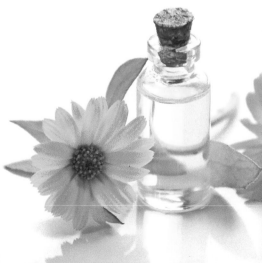

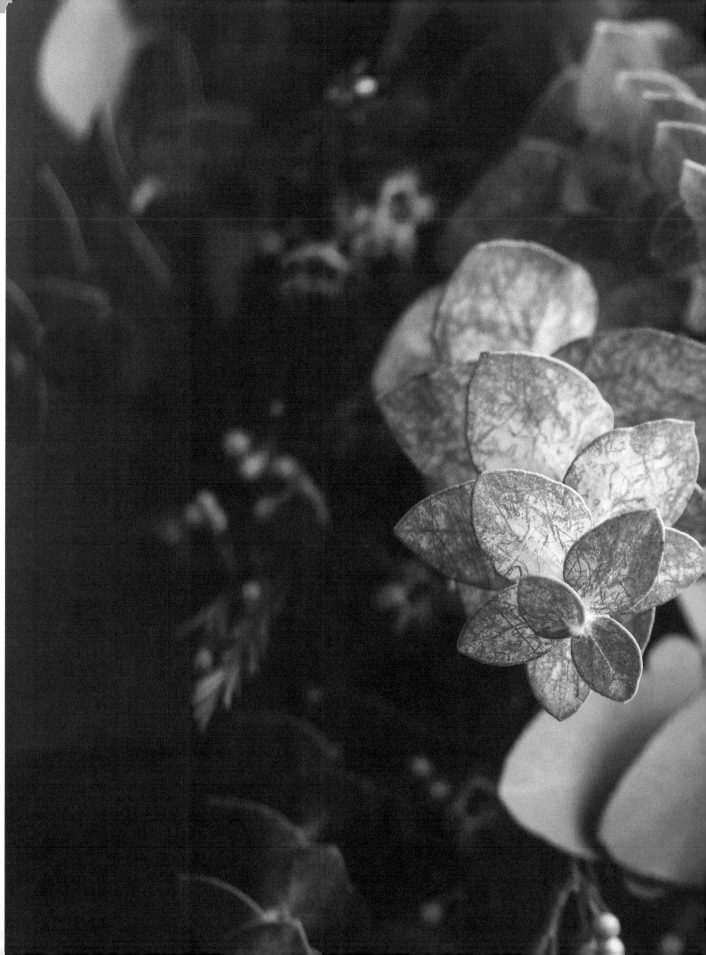

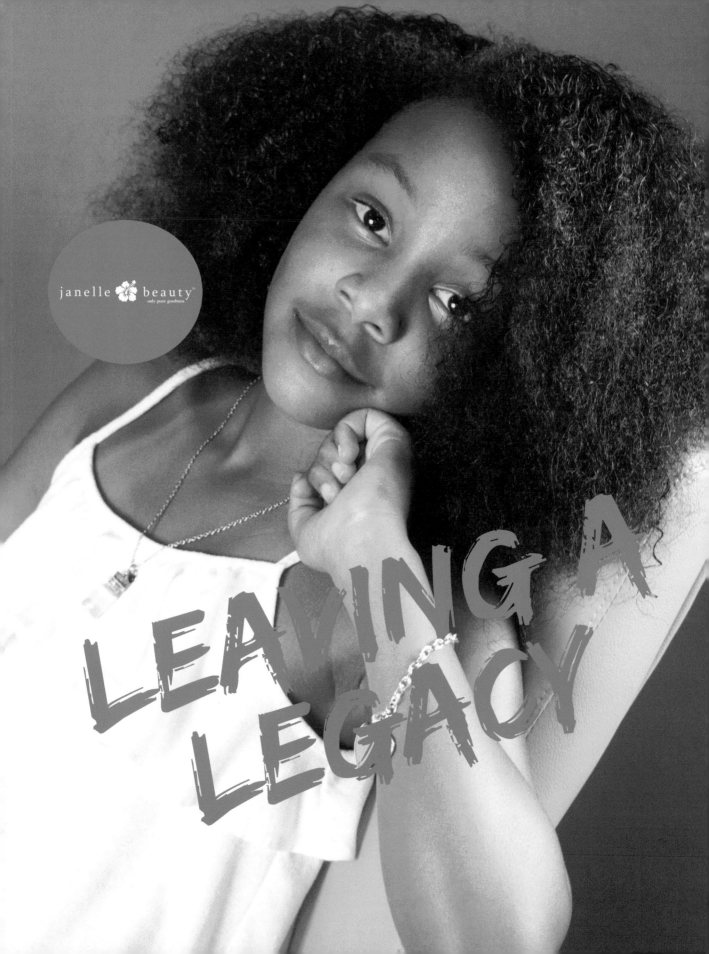

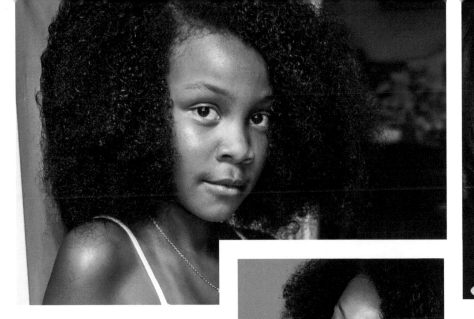

In the midst of all the upheaval at Janelle Beauty, my daughter was born. I creatively named her Janelle :)

As I watch my daughter battle the same hair struggles many girls of color endure I get inspired. I get inspired to keep making products and to keep showcasing women of color in beauty campaigns.

Representation really does matter!

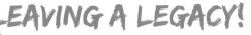

LEAVING A LEGACY!

My daughter will one day run Janelle Beauty, God-willing, and I hope to leave a legacy that she is proud of and one where she can build upon to spread beauty around the world.

My vision is for **Janelle Beauty to be a global beauty brand for women of color.** In doing so, we hope to reach the girls while they are still developing their self-image and health choices.

If you want the best and freshest beauty products the world can offer - make it yourself!
When you are ready for second best by purchasing ready made products, buy Janelle Beauty products!
Check us out at **www.janellebeauty.com**

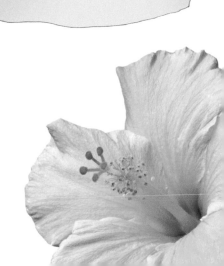

CPSIA information can be obtained
at www.ICGtesting.com
Printed in the USA
BVHW021818190820
586839BV00014B/85